Endorsements for
Breakthrough Alzheimer's Care

Breakthrough Alzheimer's Care is a wonderful blend of personal memoir and practical guidebook for caregivers. The author shows us how caregiving, though immensely hard, is a privilege when providing it for the people we love ... personal examples and stories bring richness and color that few books about caregiving provide. I have no doubt this book will provide both needed comfort and guidance for caregivers everywhere.

Nate Shinagawa, MHA, FACHE, Chief Operating Officer and Senior Vice President, University of California, Irvine (UCI) Health System

Breakthrough Alzheimer's Care is both a love story and a practical lifeline for families navigating dementia. Mark Wilson's signature optimism and heart shine through every page as he turns the overwhelming experience of caregiving into a hopeful, actionable roadmap ... [and] brings a much-needed voice to the conversation, reminding us that with compassion, leadership, and the right support, our loved ones can live not only longer, but with greater quality, dignity and joy.

Susie Singer Carter, Award Winning Filmmaker & Elder Advocate and former Alzheimer's family caregiver

The most profound gift we can offer our parents is our unwavering care and support as they confront the challenges of Alzheimer's disease and other medical hurdles. Mark Wilson's enlightening book, *Breakthrough Alzheimer's Care: A Guide to Finding Courage, Longevity, and Joy on the Journey,* stands as an indispensable companion for families embarking on this poignant journey together. This remarkable guide covers a range of crucial topics, from addressing family dynamics to fostering a team environment among healthcare professionals and carefully selecting the right caregivers to support your family.

Michele Ramos, Kathy Olsen Patient Safety Advocate, Consumer Watchdog, former Alzheimer's Family Caregiver

The title says it all! *Breakthrough Alzheimer's Care* holds within each page of each chapter vital information to help every caregiver navigate the journey, experiencing many breakthroughs and overcoming with victory.

Mark so thoroughly walks us through each challenge, each step from the first signs of Alzheimer's to the last days of your loved one's life. Mark writes from experience with passion. Mark so beautifully gave his all to care for his mom and in so doing went far and beyond to give her the best years of her life, even in her hardest season. Thank you!

Shelly Love, former Alzheimer's Family Caregiver, Alzheimer's Supports Group Leader

This is a brilliant work full of powerful advice, authenticity, vulnerability and love. There is also very helpful advice in planning for life's journey such as purchasing long term care insurance. This wonderful book serves as a toolkit and inspiration for those supporting loved ones with these conditions.

James G. Wetrich, CEO Mentor, Building Champions, Company Advisor, The Wetrich Group of Companies, Author of best seller *Stifled*

Mark Wilson has provided a compassionate overview of the journey undertaken by millions of Americans who are living with a neurodegenerative disease that causes dementia. An important offering from the unique perspective of an adult child caregiver, this is a relatable description of one family's journey. Family members are likely to see reflections of their own struggles and learn from Mr. Wilson's family's trials and successes. This book's honest sharing of one family's journey will be valuable to many.

Joshua Grill, PhD, Professor of Psychiatry & Human Behavior and Neurobiology & Behavior Director, Institute for Memory Impairments and Neurological Disorders, University of California Irvine

Mark Wilson's book, *Breakthrough Alzheimer's Care,* is a compelling resource for caregivers, healthcare professionals, and families seeking new strategies to support those living with Alzheimer's disease.

Wilson has done his research and provides practical, timely information that is vital for caregivers. His tone is personal and reassuring. He acknowledges the physical, mental, and emotional challenges of caregiving and offers practical tips for coping. His chapter summaries are especially helpful for busy caregivers who need to find information quickly.

This book is an excellent resource for those searching for a deeper understanding of the challenges of Alzheimer's care and innovative ways to provide that care with empathy and compassion.

Suzi Westmoreland, Alzheimer's Family Caregiver

What a wonderful guide!

Dr. Julie Shaw; Founder of Lead Different & Hello I'm Grieving

Millions of people live with Alzheimer's in America, and hundreds of thousands lose their lives to medical negligence every year. It is a rare gift to approach both challenges with the joy and embrace of life that shine from every page of Mark Wilson's *Breakthrough Alzheimer's Care.* Those seeking ways to advocate for their own loved ones can learn from this book.

Carmen Balber, Executive Director, ConsumerWatchdog.org

"A deeply personal and beautifully detailed account of caregiving—one that honors Mark's lived experience while offering something meaningful to anyone touched by Alzheimer's or dementia."

Lisette Diaz Santiago, Founder, MemoriGems

I came to this book as a researcher who studies memory, a designer of connection tools, and someone who has cared for loved ones with Alzheimer's. I stayed because Mark's insights go way beyond caregiving... It's the kind of book that's helpful on the first read and even more helpful when you come back to it.

Serena Lin, Neuroscience Researcher at Pomona College, Founder of the Brain Create Network, and Family Caregiver

Mark's personal stories as a caregiver son bring real heart to every page, while the Five Breakthrough Care Pillars offer a grounded, empowering framework for families. This is both a caregiving guide and a leadership journey, one that reminds us that when we care for ourselves, we show up stronger for the people we love.

Nicole Will, Founder of WillGather | WillGather Podcast, specializing in aging services, caregiver support, and senior living solutions

Breakthrough Alzheimer's Care

A Guide to Finding Courage, Longevity, and Joy

Mark Wilson

Copyeditor: Betty Lou Leaver
Cover design & layout: Opeyemi Ikuborije

ISBN: 978-1-957354-91-0
Library of Congress Control Number: 2025926063

Dedication

This book is dedicated to my mom, whose courage, spirit, and love before and during her Alzheimer's journey was and still is an inspiration to me.

This book is also dedicated to my mom's five long-term home caregivers, who with so much creativity, compassion, and love helped my mother, my sister, and me in so many wonderful and powerful ways.

I also dedicate the book to my creative, hardworking, and loving sister, who helped our remarkable caregivers and me as my co-care leader, partner, and best friend throughout Mom's Alzheimer's journey and beyond.

This is also for the hundreds of thousands of patients and their families who each year, like my mom, have suffered horribly as victims of the epidemic in this country of medical mistakes.

Finally, this book is for the tens of millions of caregivers and care leaders around the globe who work tirelessly every day to make life for their loved ones and patients with dementia a little safer, a little happier, and a little healthier each day.

CONTENTS

Acknowledgements

Thank you to the following people for helping me with the book by providing feedback, support, and encouragement, including Dina Colman Mitchell, Emil Brolick, Jill Ratliff, Christa Bourg, Tom Heetderks, Linda Scheck, Doug & Ann Armitage, Tim Galbraith, Virginia Naeve, Steve Arneson, Trisha Callella, Mackenzie Pierce, JP Elliot, Karen Kendrick, Naga Kumar, Steve Williams, Dionne Mejer, Jessie Dostis, Martin Hennessey, Jen Newans, Malia Tano, Mark Reynolds, Doug Fong, Monica Rothgery, Michele Ramos, Carmen Balber, Marina Wilson, and Claudia Mino.

Thanks as well are given to leaders throughout my career who helped positively shape my leadership know-how and experience, including Sherry Benjamins, Randy Stott, David Novak, Ed Karasek, Dennis Zeleny, Connie Colao, Peter Waller, Emil Brolick, Scott Tempel, Tim Galbraith, Steve Phillips, and John O'Keeffe

Introduction: An Empowered Alzheimer's Love Story

This book presents a step-by-step care leader's Plan to take care of your loved one with dementia. It is about life and death, joy and sadness. With Mom, I experienced great joy; I experienced sadness as well. The many small but powerful actions I took to care for Mom and how I worked to improve the impact of them during our journey together form the backbone of this book. I learned many things along the Alzheimer's Journey that Mom and I took together.

As I learned and improved each care action, they seemed to bucket into five important areas. By my continually working to achieve excellence in each of these Five Care Areas, Mom ended up living much longer than the doctors predicted—and she also seemed to live with more happiness. Does this care blueprint *cure* Alzheimer's? No, we all know there is no cure for Alzheimer's or other dementias. Alzheimer's is still a death sentence, but if we can help our loved one live longer with more joy, wouldn't we want to do that? That is exactly what I wanted to do. Having Mom with us longer with greater happiness were my two goals for leading Mom's care. Thankfully, I was able to do this.

My passion to help Mom became a leadership journey for me. Sustaining the excellence each of these five Breakthrough Care Pillars required for realizing breakthrough results took focused leadership energy on my part, and I had to both *feel* and *be* empowered in order to be a breakthrough care leader. This book, then, is a journey within a journey— an Alzheimer's care journey encompassing an empowerment journey.

How do you become an empowered care leader and how can you sustain this important leadership energy and focus over the Alzheimer's marathon? Walking each step of the empowerment journey is just as important as internalizing the five steps of a longer, healthier, and happier Alzheimer's journey. I discovered that one cannot happen without the other. So, besides sharing a love story of commitment love and sacrifice, I am sharing a story about leadership and about dissecting each of the five breakthrough care pillars I discovered. I do this so you, too, can be blessed with the gift of your loved one's greater longevity, health and joy.

The Alzheimer's and dementia research communities have been diligently seeking a cure for dementia for a long time. These smart researchers rightly want to find a medication or treatment that will cure this horrible disease. When they accomplish this, which someday they will, it will be among the greatest achievements of mankind. I do not pretend to be nearly as smart as these dedicated researchers. My approach differed significantly. Given no cure, I wanted to help Mom by taking many small actions that in the end would make a big difference for Mom's longevity, health and joy. James Clear in his bestselling book, *Atomic Habits,* describes the power of many small things coming together to make a big difference. He says it is like slowly putting a million grains of sand in a pot. At some point, the pot tips over. This was the approach I ended up taking with Mom's care. In fact, this is the only approach I could have taken with Mom since there is no cure.

I learned from my years as a human resources and leadership development executive that great results depend upon great leadership. My goal of a longer happier life for Mom would take strong leadership on my part, I believed. This book is a Leaders' Playbook for taking these many small actions that together can make a big difference for your loved one. It is a blueprint to show which of the many small but important things in dementia care collectively produce significantly greater longevity and happiness for your loved one. The Five Care Pillars represent a system: they are interrelated, interdependent, connected, and all of them are vital. If any of the Five Care Pillars are lacking or not executed at the highest level of skill, your loved one will likely not live as long as healthy or with as much joy as they potentially could. I learned in my work life that when an actual result exceeds an anticipated result by more than 40-50% percent, it is considered a "breakthrough result." Mom lived nearly three times longer than doctors expected. I could not measure her joy, but I believe if I could measure it, it would show an even greater improvement than her improvement in longevity. Even more amazing is that I believe if Mom had not been a victim of a tragic surgical mistake late in her journey (see Chapter 25), she might have lived even longer and more happily.

An Alzheimer's Love Story

Achieving excellence in these Five Important Care Areas does not happen by itself. The Care System requires a determined leader to achieve excellence in all care areas. Average longevity and happiness for dementia patients can happen with average leadership. However, breakthrough results take a passionate hands-on care leader. I chose to be the leader of Mom's care because I love my mom deeply. I knew nothing about Alzheimer's disease or Alzheimer's patient care when Mom was diagnosed with both Alzheimer's and Vascular Dementia. However, I did know I had a couple of things going for me that perhaps I could build on. First, I had great passion and drive to help Mom. She helped me so much, and I knew my love for her would give me much strength. Second, I always liked to learn new things. I thought this might help me learn what I needed to do to help Mom. And third, I had experience leading a small group of people at work. I am not unique; many dementia patients' family members share these and more skills that can help them be great care leaders of their loved one. Bolstered by these three simple assets, I dove into leading Mom's Care. Was I afraid to take on the responsibility of being Mom's care leader? Yes, but I could not think of anyone else more suited to being her care leader than me.

Everything I did to help Mom I learned on the job taking care of her. Great leaders throughout history were good learners. My hope is that this care leader's playbook to achieve Breakthrough Care results for your loved one will help you learn from my journey and give you confidence to take on the role of empowered care leader for your loved one. Both you as care leader and your loved one will have daily struggles. You will learn and travel that journey successfully together. As you lead this care system through your journey, I am hopeful and confident that you will slowly see your loved one living longer, healthier and happier because of your care leadership. The joy of seeing your loved one do better than expected will help make the struggles involved feel a little smaller. Much of the Alzheimer's journey brings heartache as you see your loved one fading. Knowing that I was helping Mom live longer, healthier, and happier more than made up for the heartache.

Mom and I shared our Alzheimer's journey day by day. As this book is our journey, it is also a deeply personal look about a family going through Alzheimer's. In this way, it is a love story about our love for each other and about how Mom was an inspiration to me to take care of her. It is a story about the hardest thing either one of us has ever done, and at the same time it is a story about the most blessed and fulfilling thing I have ever done. Like most things in life when you work very hard for something, good things often come out the other end. Mom lived longer and with more joy; and I think, very slowly, I became a slightly better version of me. This mission can make such a big difference for your loved one and for you.

Why I wrote this book

The short answer to why I wrote the book is to provide hope. There is much written about there being no cure for Alzheimer's. It is heart breaking to see our loved ones decline every day, and we miss our old life with them so very much. Given the daily challenges of dementia care, with no known cure, it is normal for families to become very discouraged and potentially paralyzed into not knowing what to do to make a positive difference in the lives of their loved one. It can be tempting, because there is little hope and no cure, to not try to do everything possible for our loved ones. I want families to know there are many positive things you can do to significantly help your loved one. I wrote this book to tell families there is hope. When you do these many small things at an excellent level, they can collectively lead to a longer, healthier, and more joyful life. I want this book to be a hope lifeline and a blueprint for action for families with loved ones with dementia.

Soon after Mom passed, I made a couple of "Spotlight on Care" podcasts for the UC Irvine's UCI MIND Alzheimer's Center on my learning from leading Mom's care at home. Listeners told me that they really liked my ideas. I kept hearing what I did for Mom was "incredible" or "wonderful." I could hear in the way listeners said those things to me that they had some doubt that they could do what I did to take care of their loved one. As I reflected on this, I thought, of course, they can do what I did. Why couldn't they do what I did? I want families to have the same wonderful experience I had taking care of Mom. I never thought taking care of her was an undue burden. It was hard, but I loved taking care of Mom and being her care leader.

Athletes who are "in the zone" maintain peak performance mode effortlessly. When I was taking care of Mom, I sometimes felt I was in "the zone." This big challenge did bring an occasional heartache, but I also experienced happiness as Mom's care leader. Caring for her became as natural to me as breathing. I worked hard, but I loved knowing I was making a big difference for someone whom I loved so much and who loved me so much. I wrote this book because I thought families and their loved ones deserve this chance to have the same gift and privilege.

I have read some very good books for families about caring for their loved one with dementia. Many of these books are excellent "how to" books on care. My goal with Mom's care surpassed just providing care; I sought to increase her longevity and infuse her days with joy.

With my career background in helping leaders grow, I want to share my leadership lessons to help you be an amazing breakthrough care leader for your loved one. I want your loved one to live healthier, happier, and longer. This is not a theoretical book or a research study. This book is my real everyday experience helping my mom. I want to inspire families to help their loved one by taking on the mission of getting breakthrough results for their loved one. If my Alzheimer's shared journey can bring hope, comfort, confidence, and results to other families, then my mom looking and smiling down from heaven will be very proud of you and be very proud of me for going all out for our loved ones.

Shifting Mindset: Is Care Leadership Right for You?

Seeing your loved one live longer with more joy can make you very happy. However, Achieving breakthrough results is challenging and requires new ways of thinking. Becoming an empowered leader of your loved one's care depends upon four important mindset shifts. *First,* changing your attitude from "I have to" to "I get to" be my loved one's care leader will put you in the right positive frame of mind to do this important work. This attitude change shifts you from thinking of care leader as being a burden to care leader being a privilege and source of joy.

Second, the mindset shift from "I am *assisting* my loved one" to "I am the *accountable leader* for all aspects of my loved one's care" takes you from aiding to leading. You cannot just be an aide to achieve breakthrough care; breakthrough care results will happen when you are a strong leader of each breakthrough care pillar. Good leaders are accountable and make things happen. The best leaders are also active, creative, and compassionate.

Third, the mindset shift changes your thinking from "how can this Alzheimer's disease be happening to me and to my loved one?" to "how can I make the biggest difference in the life of my loved one?" Of course, Alzheimer's affects you, your loved one, and your family in horrible ways; and yes, you are grieving for your old life with your loved one. The grief and loss are real, but if you get stuck in this grief or adopt the mindset of a victim, you cannot help your loved one. I am not suggesting you "stuff your feelings" or pretend you are not grieving. You need to work through your grief, but try not to get stuck in it. Later, I talk about how you can get help through this grief with individual therapy or support groups. Both therapy and support groups really helped me stay focused on Mom's care. You may have to do this personal work to get to a place where you can truly focus on being your loved one's empowered care leader. I suggest you and every single member of your Care Team will help your loved one best when all are laser focused on leading your loved one's care. This mindset shift from being a victim to being a positive empowered leader is vitally important.

Fourth, shift your mindset from "I don't know much about Alzheimer's or leading Alzheimer's care" to "no one knows more about my loved one than I, and I can learn everything I need to learn." The positive mindset combination of your knowing your loved one so well, your passion for his/her health and happiness, and your hunger to be a good learner are the final ingredients for breakthrough care leadership.

These four mindsets all have their foundation in Love. Your love for your loved one creates the path to these mindset shifts. When you are passionate and motivated and truly love your loved one, being their breakthrough care leader becomes a top priority. With this passion and love, you will figure out everything you need on your journey. If you can see yourself having or adopting these four positive mindsets, then I am confident that you will be a truly amazing care leader. This shift in how you see yourself as care leader also takes an expanded view of your own power. Expanding the view of the boundaries of your care leader job will empower you to lead in a bold way. Empowering yourself to expand your role will energize you to break through any barriers you encounter. Helping someone live happier and longer is about as noble a purpose as there is.

It is normal to find yourself getting stuck occasionally thinking about an obstacle to your being a fully empowered care leader. For example, you may still harbor a little resentment for something your loved one may have done in the past, or you may be thinking "how can I do this financially?" Later in the book I address the biggest obstacles to empowered care leadership and ways to overcome each of them. However, great care leadership starts and ends with love. With love and empowerment, you can overcome these obstacles. The rest of this book is a leaders' playbook on how to empower yourself to achieve the mission of helping your loved one live happier and hopefully longer. If I can do it, so can you!!

Care Leadership at Home or in a Community?

Taking care of your loved one at home or in a facility is a very personal decision. Many people take care of their loved one with Alzheimer's in a community setting. Most people, however, take care of their loved one for part or all their journey at home. My Alzheimer's journey with Mom was at home. I thought that with home care I would have more influence in leading Mom's Care and Mom would be happier at home. However, at the right facility, the Five Breakthrough Care Pillars can be put in place and executed very well. If you have decided that a care community is best for you and your loved one, then you can still be your loved one's breakthrough care leader, but the role will be a little different. In a facility, I would suggest you will have less direct control over your loved one's care. Your role then is to carefully observe and be sure each of the care pillars are executed at an excellent level. If you see gaps in your loved one's care, your "influence skills" will be very important in helping the facility improve care for your loved one. If the gaps are too wide or too many and/or your influence does not change the facility, I would encourage you to find a new community where the key care pillars are better executed. Your loved one will benefit, and you will also have more happiness and peace of mind.

Your Dementia Journey: Similar and Different

Mom's dementia was both Alzheimer's and Vascular Dementia. There are many types of dementia, and everyone's dementia journey is unique. Even though your journey with your loved will be different, executing The Five Breakthrough Care Pillars will be very similar. However, because everyone is a little different, before executing this care system, determine how you might need to adjust any of the components to fit your journey with your loved one. Also, before implementing the nutrition, medical, or financial recommendations in this care blueprint it may be important to check with your loved one's medical or financial advisor.

Structure of the Book

This book weaves together Mom's and my Alzheimer's experience, the Breakthrough Care Pillars, and lessons learned from my empowered care leadership. At the end of each chapter, there is a summary of the most important insights, guidelines, or tools to help you on your care leadership journey.

Since the insights and lessons in this book come from our Alzheimer's journey, I thought, for context, I should start with a little bit about Mom, the family, and me. Like your family, my family is very ordinary in many ways and very extraordinary in many other ways. A little family background will help clarify both the source of my inspiration and key events that influenced my approach to care.

After a little family background, I share the experience of getting Mom's Alzheimer's and Vascular Dementia diagnosis and how it was my call to action. Next, I share how my human resources and career experience developing leaders influenced my approach to being Mom's care leader. I outline the three leadership foundations that make for a great care leader. Next, I share what I learned about the importance of care leader self-care. Unless you as a care leader are continually reenergized and renewed, it will be impossible to sustain your essential role of care leader over the marathon. Next, I explain why a systems approach and achieving excellence in many small care pillars are important, given our brain and body's complexity. Here is an overview of the Five Breakthrough Care Pillars.

The Five Breakthrough Care Components

1. *Self-Care of the care leader is critical* to breakthrough leadership and breakthrough results for your loved one.

2. *Safety is the Gateway for the rest of the Breakthrough Care System.* Without excellence in safety foundations, you likely will never have the chance for Breakthrough longevity and happiness.

3. *Build and lead the finest Care Team for your loved one.* Your whole Care Team's mission is to bring your mission of a longer and happier life for your loved one to life.

4. *Use powerful brain/body enhancing nutrition & medications.* Many studies show how important this is.

5. *Create powerfully positively stimulating "Surround Sound" every day for your loved one.* Your loved one's total physical and emotional environment and every person encountered needs to fully reflect fun, positivity, cognitive stimulation, physical activity, familiarity, and loving comfort and care.

Concluding the first major section of the book I share the major obstacles care leaders may face and my experience of how to overcome them. The middle section of the book is dedicated to how to be an empowered care leader to execute each of the Five Breakthrough Care Pillars. The last part of the book is dedicated to the final steps of our journey.

I share what I learned in these late phases of the disease. I also address the medical surgical mistake that a doctor made directly cutting short Mom's life and how to avoid this tragic mistake. Finally, I share my grief experience and actions to help make my way through grief and onto the road of healing.

A Final Word of Encouragement before Beginning

Whether in a community or at home, making the commitment to leading your loved one's care can be scary. I was scared that I would not know enough to be responsible for Mom's care. I was also scared that I couldn't do it for as long as Mom might need care. I thought, how can I, a completely untrained person in caregiving, take better care of Mom at home than professionals can in a facility? There is a wonderful book called *Feel the Fear and Do It Anyway* by Dr. Susan Jeffers. Dr. Jeffers says it is very normal to be afraid of many things. However, the best way to overcome fear is to do the thing you are afraid of. When you walk through the fear and do something that you are afraid of, you build your self-esteem and confidence. Doing the thing you are afraid of starts a positive virtuous cycle where you gain confidence to try more things you are afraid of. That, in turn, brings you even more confidence to take even bolder actions. My journey as Mom's care leader was very much like that. One thing that most of us have going for us is that Alzheimer's or dementia usually progress slowly but unfortunately steadily. There is usually time to build care leader knowledge before the next dementia phase's challenge. I began to learn and build some confidence by trying different things in the early phases. The small actions and experiments I took helped me gain more confidence that readied me to take on the bigger challenges later in Mom's journey.

There was a point where I realized I needed help. When I was not doing all the caregiving myself, I had more time to learn and try new things that helped Mom. I was still scared, but I had more time to learn, experiment, observe the impact of care actions I took, and then refine these approaches to care.

As I learned and experimented more, the Care System began to take shape. I did not know for sure until later that it was leading to a longer happier life for Mom. I did notice however, that Mom's mood was improving. I also started getting positive compliments from Mom's neurologists that "your mom is doing remarkably well for where she is in the disease's progression." As I saw Mom grow happier and heard comments like this, I thought, "this is working, so what else can I do to make things even better." My fear lessened as I saw improvement and became inspired to work harder to provide even more creative care actions. I started to notice the actions were beginning to make a positive difference. The picture in my mind about what I needed to do slowly grew clearer.

All along the journey, fear would occasionally raise its ugly head. To help me keep my thinking positive, I would focus on the thought, "Mom always helped me in amazing ways for my whole life. Now it is my turn to help her! I will do the best I can, that's all I can do." I would ask myself, "why can't I do this?" And if I can be a good care leader for my mom, then I know you can be a great care leader for your loved one, too. This book is designed to be a blueprint so you can experience this gift, too. We may experience fear, but we can do it. anyway!

A Brief Background

Mom made it very easy to want to be the best care leader I could be. Early experiences and lessons also shaped my approach to care. These things represent the origin of my commitment, but the way Mom raised me is the biggest part of how I became her driven care leader.

Nicolena Vita Curatolo (Mom) was born in Brooklyn, New York in 1932. Mom's father, our grandfather ("Poppy") was born in Sicily and came to New York on a boat all by himself when he was 12. I would think about my grandfather coming to this country by himself as a young boy in 1901 to make a better life for his family back home. The amount of courage it took for him to overcome his fear and come to this country all by himself at that tender age inspires awe. He must have been so scared, but he did it, anyway. His courage and passion coming to this country to help his family to have a better life revealed his intense strength and drive. I often feel that whatever challenge I am facing, it can't be as hard as what Poppy did.

Mom met my dad when they lived on the same block and went to grade school together in the Bushwick section of Brooklyn New York. They started dating in High School. Italian was Mom's first language; she worked hard, learned English, and graduated from St. Joseph's Catholic College in New York. She was the first person in her family to go to college. Her passion in life was to be a teacher.

Mom and Dad married shortly after he returned from the Korean War—two young teachers in love, starting their lives together. Mom became a kindergarten teacher, and Dad a music teacher. Just nine months after they wed, they welcomed me into the world.

Mom's passion for teaching was unmistakable. Right after graduating, she began working in some of New York's most underprivileged neighborhoods, dedicating herself wholeheartedly to her students. A longtime friend and fellow teacher once told me that Mom had a kind of magic with children—she was a wonderful teacher from the very beginning.

During the first six years of my life, we lived in Brooklyn, close to both my mom's and dad's families. When I turned six, my sister Marina was born, and shortly afterward, in 1963, we packed up and moved from Brooklyn to Pomona, California.

And when I say "we," I mean *everyone*. It was a true family caravan—just like an episode of *The Beverly Hillbillies*. My grandparents, my great-aunt and great-uncle, and even my great-grandfather all made the move with us. The entire extended family relocated to Pomona at once.

After settling in Pomona Mom taught pre-school in the early days of the Head Start Program, an early childhood program for less fortunate children. Mom was exceptionally good with children, and they adored her.

Growing up with the whole family on the same block was great for me. We had Sunday dinners together. I would regularly ride my bike down the block to visit them. I always felt like a Little Prince when I went there. My friends would join me at my grandparents' house especially at lunch or dinnertime in anticipation of much delicious Italian food. My parents provided heaps of love and support. I remember how wonderful things were growing up with so much love.

In Pomona, my mom took wonderful care of me and Marina. Dad worked as the Pomona Elementary Schools travelling music teacher, where Mom was an early childhood Head Start teacher. Mom made me traditional Italian lunches to take to school. These delicious Italian lunches heightened my popularity at school. My classmates always wanted to swap meals with me, but when they asked, I would say something my grandmother sometimes would say, "nothing doing."

Mom always made every birthday and holiday special and celebratory for my sister and me and our friends. Everything mom touched was filled with fun, love, and celebration. Looking back at photos, Mom was always smiling and joyous whether she was working or taking care of her family. Mom's middle name was Vita, which means life in Italian. It certainly fit her. Throughout her life, Mom brought energy, smiles, and life to everything she did. People would always say that she would light up every room she was in with her smile.

When I was ready to enter junior high and high school, my parents wanted me to have the best education. They wanted to send me to the best junior high school (Foothill Country Day) and high school (Webb School) in the area. They both had to work multiple jobs to have enough money to send us to private school. They gracefully sacrificed to give us a wonderful education. I never remember either one complaining about the sacrifices they made for Marina and me. Even though I'm sure my mom was tired, I remember she would gladly help me with schoolwork. Whether it was grammar, vocabulary, or something else, Mom would happily drill me on my subjects.

The summer I graduated from high school, my dad got a job teaching music and conducting the orchestra at Santa Ana College. It was his dream job. Soon after, we moved closer to Dad's job at Santa Ana College in Orange County.

Mom taught pre-school and kindergarten when our family moved to Orange County. Most of Mom's time teaching in our new home in Orange County was at the Jewish School, Temple Bat Yahm. Mom was the only Christian teacher in the school and was loved by everyone there. She was like the pied piper. The kids would follow her around and loved being in her class. I watched her teach sometimes. Even though she might have 20 kids in her classroom, every child got individual attention from Mom. Every child was made by Mom to feel unique and special. That was one of Mom's talents.

Mom always built others' confidence. I remember growing up she would always tell me that whatever decision I made I would be successful. She would always say the most important thing is to be happy in what you do. I went to Law School after graduating from college. Even though

I was doing well at it, something about law school did not feel right. I was not as happy as I needed to be to do something for the rest of my life. I thought about leaving after a year and a half. It was a very hard decision because I had put a lot of time into my studies and had many student loans. Mom said it was my decision and that I would be great at whatever I decided to do. Mom got the gift of encouragement from her mother. My grandmother was the ultimate confidence builder, too. When I was afraid of a job change or some new challenge at work, I often ran it by my grandmother (we called her Nanny). Nanny would ask "has anyone else done this before?" And because someone somewhere had done whatever I was scared to do, I would say "yes, it's been done before, Nanny." Then, she would tell me that if someone else could do it, then I could do it, too. These words still motivate me today. I thought if others can write a book, then I can help others by writing a book, too. Those words of confidence have helped me with everything I have ever done in my life. I always felt so loved and supported by Mom, Dad, Nanny, and the entire family.

In 1989, Dad passed away. He died when he was just 56 with a cancerous brain tumor. From diagnosis to his death was less than 90 days. Very soon after Dad passed, I was approached by an insurance agent who asked me if I wanted to buy long term-care insurance for my mom. I did not know what it was, and I did not know anyone who had it. God blessed me that day because I decided to purchase it for Mom. I will discuss the importance of long-term care insurance and the types of long-term care insurance policies in Chapter 5. For now, let me say buying long-term care insurance for my mom was by far the best financial decision I've made.

The shock of my dad's unexpected death was devastating for all of us, especially Mom. It took a while for Mom to get over the heartbreak of losing her childhood sweetheart. Mom eventually went back to work at the same Temple School. Mom had lots of friends who helped her get through this dark period of losing Dad. My wonderful and always positive grandmother, and Mom's friends at her school and at our church were critical to helping my mom work her way through her grief. Mom's love and magnetism always drew wonderful people into her life who supported her well.

Mom and I were always great friends. My dad's passing brought us all even closer. I became even closer to Mom and my sister Marina. Mom got her infectious enthusiasm and joy back after a very long time grieving for my dad.

Another caregiving lesson came my way a few years later when my loving grandmother was diagnosed with older age leukemia. This is a very slow-moving leukemia. She was 91, but spry, energetic, and clear headed. Nanny and I had always looked out for each other. I started taking her to her weekly outpatient infusion treatment. Like Mom, Nanny was a very strong Sicilian woman.

As I began to help my grandmother through leukemia, I learned things that helped me help Mom later through her Alzheimer's journey. I have lots of wonderful Nanny memories. One having to do with medical care is about holding healthcare workers to high standards. In Sicily when someone was not very good at a job, they would be called a "shoemaker." One day Nanny and I were in the waiting room at the leukemia infusion center. She leaned over to me and whispered, "don't let that shoemaker take care of me." When the medical technician did Nanny's infusions, he would often hurt her. He would have to poke her several times before he found the vein. I leaned over to her and said, "Don't worry, Nanny; I won't let him do your infusions anymore." I insisted someone else do her infusions from that day forward. I learned that there is no reason anyone should accept less than the best care. You don't need to tolerate a "shoemaker" taking care of your loved one. I apologize if I offended any shoemakers who may be reading this book.

The second major medical learning from these early years was the challenge of being in an HMO. My grandmother was in a Medicare HMO (now euphemistically called Medicare Advantage). We always experienced delay and encountered bureaucratic obstacles in getting Nanny the needed approvals to see the desired specialists. To avoid these hurdles, I made sure Mom was on regular Medicare and a Medicare

Supplement. We then could go to any physician we wanted at any time we wanted. For Mom, then, I was able to find the best doctors more quickly and more easily fire any doctors we did not like.

The third medical care lesson I learned from my experience helping Nanny was in 2005. My grandmother took a fall that put her in the hospital. She was quickly shuffled into a "rehab facility." I frequently visited her in the facility. Often, she needed something simple like help going to the bathroom, and no one was around to help her.

After a month, I moved Nanny to a different, supposedly better, facility, but the care was essentially the same. I was so frustrated that nobody was able to take care of Nanny when she needed help. The facility did not have enough caregivers. The ratio of medical staff to patients was insufficient. I would have medical questions, and it was impossible to get answers when I needed them. After a month in this second facility, Nanny got sepsis and died. The sepsis was from a urinary tract infection from having to wait to be cleaned or having to hold it too long. These two rehab facilities were loaded with shoemakers.

After this caregiving experience, I was determined that any loved one over which I had any influence would not go to a facility but rather be taken care of at home. I had no idea how I would do that, but even at that time, I knew there must be a way. Like Mom used to say, "Where there is a will, there is a way." Like most people, I assumed since my grandmother needed physical therapy for a fall, she needed to go to a rehab facility. I later learned while caring for my mom that this is not necessarily true. I learned that one can get any kind of medical, professional, physical therapy, respiratory therapy, speech therapy, caregivers, RNs, and even medical doctors all in your home. Also, if you have core Medicare and a Medicare supplement all these medical specialists and services will be completely paid for in your home. I'm not sure if many of today's Medicare Advantage policies would pay for all your home providers of medical services; that is something that each individual family would need to look into. However, Core Medicare does. I learned that it is not that hard to make your home a better and more comfortable "rehab" place than a rehab facility.

I loved my grandmother immensely. We had lots of fun, and she was my best friend. She had a very positive influence on me. She worked hard her whole life. She believed there is nothing you cannot do if you put your mind to it and work hard. Like Mom, she believed in people and assumed the best in them. Mom was brave, smart, kind, and the most loving person I have ever known. I still talk about and miss Nanny and Mom every single day.

You see what a wonderful family I have? Many of you have similar family stories about sacrifice and love. I learned so much from my family and am so proud of them. It should be no surprise that it was very natural for me to become a passionate care leader for Mom. Tapping into the strength of your family background and its love and sacrifice may be a motivational force for you as well.

Beginning an Empowered

Care Leader's Journey

CHAPTER 1

Denial and Diagnosis:
Shock and Call to Action

With that little bit of family background under your belt, it is time for me to begin sharing our Alzheimer's journey and the blueprint for leading breakthrough care.

How did our Alzheimer's journey start? Increasingly I noticed that Mom was forgetting things and repeating herself. Basic things she had done with grace and ease were becoming harder for her. She was showing signs that something was different. I thought Mom, at age 75, was just experiencing age-appopriate forgetfulness. I was in denial. My sister Marina insisted that we get Mom formally tested, and I'm very glad she pushed me. We went to one of the best Alzheimer's Centers in the country: UCI MIND in Irvine, California. After scans, blood tests, and cognitive testing, we received the diagnosis that my mom suffered from both Alzheimer's and Vascular Dementia. There are many kinds of dementias including Lewy Body, Vascular, Frontal Lobe, and others. Alzheimer's is the most common type. These specific types of dementias and causes differ. The behavioral symptoms are a little different by type and can even vary somewhat by person. Even though Mom's Alzheimer's journey is unique, our journey is very likely more similar than different from what you and your loved one will experience.

Getting any dementia diagnosis is very difficult for families. There is often denial, and the patient or family doesn't want to go through the testing. If you are not sure if your loved one has Alzheimer's or another form of dementia, you can get a general idea by looking at one of the many lists of comparative behaviors that are readily available. Most describe the differences between normal aging and Alzheimer's or other form of dementia. I share one such list in this chapter's summary. If your loved one resists testing, you can confirm it is enjoyable. The cognitive testing is fun, with puzzles, and pictures. You also can say you would really like them tested because you really care about them and their health. It is helpful to get a formal medical diagnosis. This will help get you on the right medical path for care.

Mom's formal medical diagnosis was in 2007. The neurologist at UCI MIND told my sister and me that, based on Mom being in her mid-seventies and the stage of Alzheimer's and Vascular dementia she was in, it is likely that Mom would live roughly five more years. Five years!! We were in shock! I went from denial to shock and then sadness almost immediately.

After reeling from this prognosis, we asked the neurologist what we should do. She immediately put Mom on Aricept, and very soon after that, Mom was put on Namenda. These two classes of drugs were the FDA approved drugs at the time used to slow the progression of this disease. Even though some newer drugs are starting to show some promise in slowing dementia, these are still the two core go-to medications for anyone diagnosed with dementia. Unfortunately, there is still no cure for this horrible disease.

After reflecting on Mom's diagnosis, my mind started reeling. I felt scared, and panic set in. I did not know anything about Alzheimer's, but I knew this diagnosis was not good. I quickly read everything I could about the disease. I also spoke with the local Alzheimer's Association about Mom's symptoms and asked for tips about caring for her. I was a sponge, soaking up all I could about the disease and the associated care. I learned about the power of good nutrition, physical movement, and a positive, fun, stimulating, and loving environment for Alzheimer's patients. I learned about the phases of the Alzheimer's journey. I also started learning about home safety and communicating effectively with Alzheimer's patients. I thought that Mom would be better off at home if

I could figure out how to do home care well. I am so glad our wonderful neurologist was so direct in telling us she thought Mom would only live for roughly five more years. It spurred me to action. I began thinking to myself, "I am going to prove this wonderful and caring doctor wrong. I am going to figure out how Mom will live longer than five years!" I did not know how I was going to do this or whether it was even possible. But, by God, I was going to try. I thought that I was going to do my very best to make her Alzheimer's journey the longest, healthiest, and happiest Alzheimer's journey ever. I was determined. Our terrific neurologist's prognosis gave me the spur to act and to act boldly.

Chapter Summary

1. It is very easy to be in denial about your loved one's dementia. It is also very hard for families to take the step to get your loved one tested and diagnosed.

2. It is important to know if your loved one has Alzheimer's or another dementia. The sooner you get started on the medications, cognitive enhancing nutrition, a stimulating environment, a plan to keep your loved one moving and active, and planning overall for the journey the better off you and they will be.

3. If you or your loved one is afraid of doing the testing, don't frame the testing as scary. Keep the idea of testing fun, exciting, positive, and important. The cognitive part of the testing can be seen as fun. Frame the testing as a normal way to see how your loved one is doing and how to keep them healthy.

4. If you get the diagnosis of dementia, try not to be depressed or paralyzed. Try to use it as a call to action to begin putting a plan in place and taking bold action to help your loved one.

Is It Normal Aging or Dementia?

Normal Aging

- unable to remember details of a conversation or event a year ago
- unable to remember the name of an acquaintance
- unable to remember things or events on occasion
- worried about memory (but friends and relatives are not)

Signs of Dementia

- unable to recall details of a very recent conversation
- can't recognize or doesn't know the names of family members
- frequently forgets things or events
- has frequent pauses where the right words cannot be found
- friends and family have noticed and are worried

CHAPTER 2

Many Small Changes Make a Big Difference: Case for a Care System

The definition of a *system* is a set of things working together as parts of an interconnected network. Medical researchers say that the brain is one of the most complex systems we know. The brain has more connections than there are stars in the galaxies. There are over 100 billion neurons and many trillions of synapse connections. This complexity is awe-inspiring. Our brain can do many amazing things. It is a wonderful blessing and can sometimes be a bit of a curse. Our brain is one of the most unknown and important frontiers.

There is no medicine or operation that can definitively cure Alzheimer's. Despite the plot of two of my favorite movies, Mel Brook's *Young Frankenstein*, a funny parody of Frankenstein, and Steve Martin's The *Man with Two Brains,* a funny movie about a neurologist who has invented a way to transplant brains by simply screwing off the top of one's head ("The Cranial Screw Top Method"), unlike other organs due to its complexity the brain cannot be transplanted. Because of the brain's complexity, many different triggers can interact and cause dementia. We struggle with research because there are so many different health conditions that can have an impact on dementia. Some of these include infection, injury, nutritional deficiency, heart health, certain medications, long-term metabolic dysfunction, viruses, and exposure to harmful chemicals, among others. Knowledge of the brain is growing rapidly, but there is so much we still don't know. If you're interested in a deeper look at the medical science of dementia, I suggest reading Dr. Sanjay Gupta's book *Keep Sharp: Build a Better Brain at any Age* (2021). It is a terrific book on the science of dementia and also provides a roadmap to help minimize your risk of getting dementia. This book reminds us of how much we know and don't know about dementias and their possible causes.

Due to our brain's complexity, it is very difficult to know the exact cause and effect of dementia and therefore what exactly triggers the dementia or how best to manage it. This makes it extremely challenging to develop a single medicine to cure Alzheimer's and other dementias. Today, there is no silver bullet cure. There are, however, actions to take that collectively have a high correlation to brain health. As Dr. Gupta and others are discovering, there are many things we can do. Studies also are beginning to show that many of the things that reduce the risk of getting dementia can also slow down the symptoms for those who do have it. There may not be a silver bullet, but there is hope for dementia patients. It seems that doing many small things that have a small amount of evidence of improving brain and physical health collectively can make a big difference.

After Mom's diagnosis, I learned as much as possible about all these small things that might lead to an improvement for Mom. I thought that if I could do as many of these things as possible, I could help her in her Alzheimer's journey. I thought as long as I was not harming Mom, why not do lots of small things to help her. My approach made sense to me and eventually seemed to work. Can I prove what specific action caused what benefit? No, I cannot; however, I did observe very positive results. Many small things coming together created a powerful interconnected system for improvement. Mom's Alzheimer's slowed, and she lived much longer and much happier because of this system.

Chapter Summary

1. The human brain is among the most complex system on the planet; there are billions of interconnected neurons. This overwhelming complexity is why dementia has thus far not been cured with medication.

2. There are so many things we don't know about the brain. However, we do know about things that help the brain function. These include brain healthy nutrition, mobility, exercise, cognitive stimulation, social connections, positivity, and good physical health with an absence of diseases like high blood pressure, heart problems, or diabetes.

3. At this stage of what we know about the brain, the best that loving families can do is to implement as many of these small benefit ideas as we can. All these simultaneous brain-and-body-enhancing actions I found worked together to indeed create greater health, happiness, and longevity. Greater health, longevity, and happiness is the mission of the Breakthrough Dementia Care System.

The Five Breakthrough Pillars

The traditional linear approach to scientific research involves isolating factors and determining the impact one factor at a time. Given the vast complexity of the brain, this research method makes progress toward a cure very slow.

Many leaders in the field, whether pharmaceutical, nutritional, or lifestyle, have numerous excellent ideas that can help with brain health. Even though some of these ideas may not have gone through the rigorous scientific method the FDA requires for a pharmaceutical drug, there is at least some evidence to support all the things that I tried for Mom. Because there is no cure for the disease and because the disease will lead to certain death, I felt why not try all these things. If I found something that appeared helpful and did not hurt Mom, I included it in the system.

Because of the way we prove medical solutions, it is impossible to know how many of these small actions are really needed to create a big difference. Our loved ones with this disease don't have time to wait for a cure. As the leader of your loved one's care, you have a unique and special opportunity to weave together these ideas into a Breakthrough Care System for your loved one. I will detail in later chapters how to lead the implementation of each pillar of the Breakthrough Care System and how your leadership is vitally important to create the excellence required for each.

The Five Breakthrough Pillars

1. *Self-Care is the Care Leader's Source of Renewable Energy* to sustain breakthrough care leadership. Without you, the energized care leader, very little that is "breakthrough" is going to happen for your loved one.

2. *Safety is the Gateway to Breakthrough.* If your loved one is not safe, there is little you can do that will help them. Your loved one will not live longer, healthier, or happier if they are not safe.

3. *Build and Lead the Finest Care Team Ever.* Ensure the whole team is tenaciously focused on executing all the breakthrough pillars at the highest level. Without the finest care team, this level of care will not be sustainable. Your Care Team, working through you, the leader, brings Breakthrough Care to life.

4. *Use Powerful Brain/Body-Enhancing Nutrition & Medications.* These nutrients can lead to a better mind and better health overall. Brain and physical health are connected systems. With a healthier brain and good physical health, your loved one can live longer and happier.

5. *Fill Your Loved One's World with Fun, Love, Compassion, Stimulation, and Familiarity: Environment & People.* Create Surround Sound for your loved one so every aspect of their physical environment and every person they encounter, every day, are full of fun, cognitive and physical stimulation, compassionate love, and are familiar. Make sure your loved one feels positivity, stimulation, caring, and familiar love from everyone and everything every single day.

You may notice that these breakthrough care pillars touch on a broad range of things that contribute to overall physical health, brain health, and emotional health. Physical health, brain and mental health, positivity, and love all work together. Everyone on Team Mom became crystal clear that their mission was to help Mom at the highest level for each one of these care pillars.

In creating the Breakthrough Care System, I learned from the best caregivers and best medical professionals. I watched and learned what the best of our Caregivers did. I started codifying what worked and then tried to communicate the best ideas across the team.

As you see improvement, I believe it is possible to actually enjoy being your loved one's care leader. If your loved one is in a facility, I am confident you can use your empowered influence to make sure each of these Breakthrough Care Pillars are being executed in the facility at the highest level.

Dementia is an unbelievably challenging journey. It can be by far the hardest experience your loved one and you will ever face. I hope leading these Five Breakthrough Pillars will be positively transformative for your loved one and for you. In the following chapters, I will share my experience and the details in leading all five areas and how they helped Mom. Much of the difference is up to you as care leader! Remember my grandmother's advice I shared with you, "if it has been done before, you can do it, too" so if I can do this, so can you! Like Mom would often say, "if there is a will there is a way." So, if your will is high enough, you can do this!

Chapter Summary

1. Each of the Five Breakthrough Care Pillars requires leadership. The care leader needs to ensure execution of all five of these at the highest level. Without self-care, you, the care leader, will lose the necessary energy to sustain the marathon that is dementia care leadership.

2. A long-term outstanding care team is crucial for breakthrough results. If your loved one is not safe, not continually stimulated, not getting the best medical care, not getting the very best nutrition, mobility, love, or any other element is lacking, the

system will not create breakthrough results. All these small improvements work together for big results.

3. Your outstanding care team brings the breakthrough pillars to life. However, you will not find these outstanding team members or lead them to continuously improve care without your strong leadership. The care leader works through a powerful care team to bring the Breakthrough Care System to life.

CHAPTER 4

The Foundation for Empowered Care Leaders

Since leading breakthrough care is first about being a strong leader, I thought I would share three simple but important foundational characteristics of great leaders. Outstanding leaders in all walks of life have always had these three common foundational leadership characteristics: (1) a passion to lead; (2) a commitment to building know-how in their field; and (3) the drive to build and lead a mission-aligned championship team.

I knew I had to tap into these three leadership foundational characteristics to truly help Mom. I may have been naïve, but I thought with a passion and drive for helping Mom and for learning, I could lead Mom's care. The very first step to being an empowered care leader was to see myself as Mom's care leader. Getting a breakthrough result in any field takes a passionate and active leader to bring everything together to achieve the mission they are passionate about.

Real Passion to Lead Your Loved One's Care

To be the care leader that Mom deserved, I first had to find my passion to do this. I found my passion in several places. First, my passion came from my deep love and commitment to Mom. Mom had made many difficult sacrifices over a long period of time to help my sister and me have a better life. Mom worked at being a great teacher and even harder at being a caring and loving mother. I was committed to her because she was so committed to us. For me, sacrificing for the people you love and who love you is as natural as breathing.

Second, my passion came from feeling I was blessed; I felt this was the right thing to do. My friends and family marveled at the personal sacrifices I made to take care of Mom. Taking care of Mom did not feel like sacrifice. I had no question that what I was doing was the right thing. Love is sacrifice. Mothers and fathers sacrifice for their children all the time. Sacrifices are made for family. Most faiths place sacrifice at the core of their faith. We know Jesus made the ultimate sacrifice. God gives us the gifts of forgiveness, love, and sacrifice. My passion to lead, therefore, also came partly from my faith and hope in God. Mathew Kelly, a wonderful Catholic writer, and speaker talks about "holy moments" in his wonderful book called *Holy Moments* (2022). A Holy Moment he says come most often from helping others, inspired by the gift of God's love. I believe my decision to leave my successful executive career to fully commit to taking care of Mom was such a Holy Moment. Yes, there was some economic and personal fear in my decision, but there was also no doubt it was the right decision. Our money and talents are meant to support and align with our deepest values. Giving my mom the longest and best life possible was the highest value and best use of my time and my financial resources. I found I had many of these Holy Moments along the path of our Alzheimer's journey together.

The third source of my passion to lead mom's care comes from the inspiration and the role-modelling gift I received from my ancestors. My grandparents, who were Italian immigrants, made many sacrifices to make a better life for the family. Sacrifice for family and for a higher purpose is in my DNA, and I found for me is also very natural and life affirming.

In my leadership development work experience. I found the best leaders had an unparalleled passion for their mission or goal. My crystal-clear mission with Mom was to help her live longer and happier. To sustain the mental, emotional, and physical energy needed to be an Alzheimer's care leader, it takes that kind of crystal-clear mission, and it also takes resilience. Resilience is the ability to bounce back in the face of challenge, disappointment, and adversity. Alzheimer's care has lots of need for resilience. The passion for my mission for Mom's longer and happier life, along with self-care helped me be resilient. My deep love for Mom, my faith and sense of what is right that Mom instilled in me, and a family history of sacrificing for what's important were the fuel that kept me energized as care leader.

Building Knowledge about Dementia and Dementia Care

Soon after Mom was diagnosed, she needed more than just casual care, so I realized I needed to help her more and learn a lot more about care. Soon after, I decided to leave the workplace to take care of Mom full-time at home. My learning quest began.

I learned the blocking and tackling of taking care of an Alzheimer's patient. First, there was learning about safety fundamentals, like safe walking and safe bathing. Second, I learned about communicating effectively with an Alzheimer's patient when they are agitated or confused. I also read and learned alternative approaches to help Alzheimer's patients. These included cognitive stimulation with puzzles, art, and music. It included an Alzheimer's friendly diet, supplements, physical movement, as well as creating an environment that was familiar, fun, and especially loving. I needed to get moving to help Mom with all these things; and I needed to do it quickly. In the resources section of this book, I include many of these references in my learning journey.

I experienced a steep learning curve to discover all about Alzheimer's disease, caregiving, new studies, and methods of helping dementia patients, as well as to locate resources. I read as many books and articles on Alzheimer's care as I could. I spoke to caregiving Agencies, medical specialists, and others. I had a real hunger to know what I could do to slow down Mom's disease and make her happier. I was learning from the moment of my mom's diagnosis throughout our entire Alzheimer's journey. I continually experimented to improve Mom's care. When I thought some aspect of care needed to be added, refined, or eliminated, I did it.

Whether you are leading your loved one's care or are a new CEO of a company, the best leaders realize that they must learn all about their new role and the relevant subject matter to accomplish their important mission. There is nothing embarrassing about having to learn a lot; learning is part of the privilege of leadership. Being your loved one's breakthrough care leader is a privilege, a gift, and more doable than you might think.

Building and Leading a Championship Care Team

In my human resources life, I tried to help leaders improve their results and achieve success as well as their dreams. This was mostly achieved through the help of others. The third characteristic of all great leaders is to build a championship team in support of their mission. By late 2012, Mom needed more help than Marina and I could provide. I was getting very little sleep, and I began to realize I was not able to provide the exceptional care I wanted. I was also not having enough time to find all the innovative ways to extend Mom's life and happiness. Good leaders know they cannot accomplish their mission by themselves; I thought Mom would be much better off if I could build a championship care team around me that would help me help her at a higher level.

The best leaders know how to lead a team of great people, singularly focused, on their mission. Leaders achieve their breakthrough results through their teams. These leaders usually guide specialists that have more knowledge than they have in that specialty. Even though the leader may not have as much knowledge as their specialist team, the leader usually has the clearest vision of the mission. Leaders are also great at hiring smart and capable people and then retaining and motivating them to accomplish the mission. These great leaders are willing to hire the best, coach for excellence, and let go of those who are less competent or don't have the needed passion for the mission.

My mission of creating the most positive Alzheimer's experience for Mom leading to a longer and more joyful Alzheimer's journey was a "stretch goal." A "stretch goal" is a goal that is almost out of reach but still achievable. A stretch goal stretches you as leader and stretches your team. To achieve a stretch goal, you and your team need to work harder and more creatively. Since there is no cure for Alzheimer's, the mission of Mom living a longer and a happier life was clearly a stretch goal. Great leaders know that setting a stretch goal helps get the very best from them and their team. The core idea with stretch goals is that if you do not expect much you won't get much. As I shifted my care leadership role away from doing most of the direct care, the quality of my Care Team became everything. Every single member of Mom's care team had to be the best and, at the same time, have the same tremendous passion that I had for my mission with Mom.

There are several teams that I ended up leading for Team Mom. First, I led a team of personal direct caregivers. Direct caregivers are the people who provide the hands-on care Mom needed every day. As the disease progressed, I needed more direct care. During the last six years, Mom needed 24-hour care including safe and enjoyable bathing, dressing, help walking, and making sure she was eating safely. These direct caregivers also led the "magic elements." The magic, less tangible but hugely important, includes connecting with Mom, having fun, stimulating her creativity and cognition, providing creative mobility activities, and giving her lots of love and attention. Because finding caregivers capable of magic was so important, I saw the home care agencies, who helped me find incredible direct caregivers, as a very important part of Team Mom.

Second, I became the leader of Mom's physicians' team. The core of Mom's doctor team consisted of a neurologist specializing in Alzheimer's and Mom's primary doctor. Because Mom had some additional medical issues, the medical specialties team also eventually included a cardiologist, a pulmonologist, a dermatologist, and a urologist.

Finally, I led other specialists on Team Mom. Other members included a regular at- home dentist, an at-home physical therapist, an at- home podiatrist, and at-home hair care. Later, I will share the mindset and tips on leading all these other specialists' teams for Mom.

These doctors and other specialists were a key part of Mom's team because without great medical and other important care, Mom would not be very healthy or happy. I found it important to view each of these specialized and independent professionals as "team members" of Mom's care team. Even though all of them were independent and specialized, I had to think of them as working for me and Team Mom. They helped me provide Breakthrough Care. If any doctor, caregiver, or other specialist was not performing to their peak ability and demonstrating compassionate care and creativity for Mom, they could not be on Team Mom.

I had very high standards of excellence for every member of my mom's care team. There is a simple and practical leadership tool I learned working in human resources that can help gauge the level of commitment of you or of any one on your care team. It is called the Accountability Ladder. A great leader needs to be high on the Accountability Ladder. The higher rungs on the ladder are "own it," "find solutions," and "make it happen." The lowest, or "victim," rungs of the accountability ladder are "unaware," "blame others," "find excuses," and "wait and hope." I wanted to be high on the Accountability Ladder, and I needed everyone on Team Mom to be on the high rungs of the ladder, too. I could not just "wait and hope" Mom's care team members were good enough to help Mom. If you have a clear mission, a vision of greatness, and clear expectations, if a team member is basically strong, then you can coach a care team member to go from good to great. If after some coaching performance did not improve, I would find a replacement for that team member. This was true for caregivers, physicians, or anyone else on Team Mom. The mission was too important not to act quickly. Every single member of Mom's care team was critical for her and an essential part of Mom's Breakthrough Care System. I could not afford a single weak link. My home care agencies sourced great caregivers, and I learned how to find and research excellent medical and other specialists. There are many caregivers, physicians, and other providers to choose from; there is no need to tolerate less than stellar care for your loved one. With Alzheimer's, there is no time to wait; it helps to act quickly to find, motivate, and keep the best care for your loved one. Stay on the empowered top rungs of the "Accountability Ladder" for the best results.

Chapter Summary

The three breakthrough care leadership foundations are all important and mutually reinforcing. The passion to lead and the passion for mission drives you to learn what you need to do to help your loved one and to find and lead the best team to implement the live-longer-and-happier dementia mission. The three foundations work together for breakthrough. John O'Keeffe is a leading consultant on how leaders create game changing or frame breaking results. A very important part of being a breakthrough leader, he says, starts with identifying and overcoming mindsets that limit you. Is your confidence limiting you? Is hearing "there is no cure for Alzheimer's" discouraging or limiting you?" In Chapter 5, I share some more of these limiting mindsets and obstacles and how best to overcome them.

By tapping into your deep passion to help your loved one and your ability to learn, you can be a breakthrough care leader of the very best care team for your loved one. You can make a huge difference in their life and in yours.

1. The Three Breakthrough Care Leader Foundations are:

    a. Have a real passion to lead your loved one's care.

    b. Build knowledge about dementia & dementia care.

    c. Build and lead a championship care team for your loved one.

2. It is normal to feel a little shaky on these foundations, but if you have passion to help your loved one, you can learn these things. Being high on the Accountability Ladder and not on the "victim" or "wait and hope" rung energized me to do what I needed to be Mom's care leader. When you are high on the Accountability Ladder you can learn to be Breakthrough Leader.

    The following reflection questions point to how you can bolster these important care leader foundations.

The Readiness Checklist for the Empowered Care Leader

Readiness: Passion to Lead Your Loved One's Care

1. How strong is your passion to lead your loved one's care?

    a. Do you have issues that are obstacles to your commitment? (See Ch. 5 on Overcoming the Four Obstacles to care leadership to help on this)

    b. How are your faith and trust in God or Higher Power?

    You will likely at some point on the journey need to call on your faith for continued strength and resilience. When you pray for strength, you may hear your calling.

    c. Do you usually take responsibility for things, or do you simply hope things will get better? Do you tend to blame others when things go wrong? If you tend to see yourself as a victim, know that you are more powerful than you see yourself. Reflect on all the hard things you have successfully done in your life; these will help you feel the empowerment you have earned.

    d. Do you believe that if you work hard enough on something, you will be successful? You have probably been very successful in many areas of your life; get in touch with those things to feel more empowered.

    e. How much time can you commit to leading your loved one's care? If your time appears limited, how can you commit more time? (Time is a potential obstacle; See Ch. 5 on Overcoming Time Obstacles)

    f. How willing are you to make a financial sacrifice for your loved one's care? There are many things that can be done to help here (See Ch. 5 on Overcoming the Financial Obstacle)

Readiness: Build Knowledge about Dementia and Dementia Care

How strong is your curiosity to learn new things, especially when they are important to you?

a. Do you like to learn?

b. Are you relatively comfortable experimenting with new things and then improving them as you go?

c. Are you comfortable with ambiguity? Do you require a clear path before you take on a new task or challenge?

You probably have learned lots of important things in your life whether they are in school or in the workplace. If you had a passion for something you put in the time and energy to learn it. Let this past learning be an inspiration to this new learning challenge with your loved one.

Readiness: Build and Lead a Championship Care Team

What is your comfort in leading others toward a mission? Note: you don't have to have had formal experience leading a team to be good at leading others.

a. Are you willing to tell others what you expect from them?

b. Are you good at giving praise or recognition when someone does something well?

c. Are you willing to let people know that they have not met your expectations?

d. Are you willing to coach others? If that person does not improve after your coaching, can you see yourself replacing them?

e. Could you see yourself striking the balance between creating an environment of recognition, fun, and love while also being clear that what someone is doing is seriously important and that you have high expectations of them.

You may not have formally led a team at work, but the chances are you have led your family and/or friends, or maybe you have led volunteers for a charity or have other leadership experiences. In the corporate world, I have seen people step into leadership roles with no experience who quickly did a remarkable job leading their team. If your drive for the mission is high and you are willing to learn, you can be an incredible leader without prior leadership experience.

As you think about your overall readiness to be care leader for your loved one, if you feel you have gaps, don't be discouraged. I had many areas to work on when I decided to be Mom's care leader. If your passion and urgency to help your loved one is strong, you will overcome any shortcomings. Seek help from people you know who may be strong in the areas where you may need a little bolstering. Knowing the importance of your mission to help your loved one, people will be glad to help you. Also, in the resources section at the end of the book, I include many resources to help you in these leadership foundation areas.

CHAPTER 5

Overcoming Obstacles to Empowered Care Leadership

As you think about embarking on your breakthrough dementia journey with your loved one, here are the four most common obstacles a loved one's care leader might face and the ways to work to overcome each of the four obstacles.

Overcoming the Psychological Obstacle

The first psychological obstacle to care leadership is that there could be some baggage from your past. You may have past resentments that could be getting in the way of being fully committed to being your loved one's care leader. There may be past conflicts in which your loved one did not treat you the way you thought you should be treated. There could also be some family dynamics involving siblings who aren't helping you or helping your loved one.

There is a wonderful book by Patti Davis (2021) called *Floating in The Deep End*. The author talks about all kinds of great things she learned taking care of her father. The part that stood out for me was how she overcame past resentments to become an outstanding care leader for her father, Ronald Reagan, in his Alzheimer's journey. The short answer to help someone to overcome past resentments is to move away from being stuck in the past, move toward being an adult, and be grateful that you can choose love. Love is important for a fulfilled life. Your loved one's life is on the line with dementia; there is no time to wait to have a loving relationship with your loved one. Now is the time to try to be the best person you can be. Be the adult and break through your resentments because your loved one needs you now more than ever.

Even though I was fortunate that I did not have these past resentments taking care of Mom and had excellent family support from my sister, when I was deep into leading Mom's care, I found a therapist who really helped me with the psychological and emotional challenges of seeing Mom in a slow and devastating decline over such a long period of time. A therapist or support group that focuses on the psychological challenges of seeing your loved one in decline and its associated grief, or on past resentments, can really help you with these emotional challenges. My therapist helped me focus on the positive and wonderful things about Mom as well as to know that the grief from slowly losing someone you love is very normal. I wanted to be a strong and positive leader for Mom and my care team; this psychological support was important for my strength and resilience. My sessions with the therapist were my private time to share and vent and get good advice. If I had stuffed or buried these feelings, I would not have been as good a care leader as Mom deserved. I also avoided what happened when my dad died, where because I did not work through the feelings I ended up with medical issues from the internalized stress.

My hope is that you will rise above any psychological obstacles and have the spirit of forgiveness and love. When you decide to make a loved based sacrifice and forgive resentments, you can be open to taking care of your loved one with more peace, energy, and grace. You then can be free to embrace and experience a blessed and special friendship in your dementia journey with your loved one.

Overcoming the Financial Obstacle

Alzheimer's and other dementia care is very expensive whether that care is at home or in a facility. Your loved one at some point will need a great deal of medical and other care. Your cherished one will at some point need hands-on care for things like walking, eating, and other daily activities. Unfortunately, Alzheimer's slowly takes away all of the patients' ability to take care of themselves.

The best thing you can do for your loved one is to purchase a long-term insurance policy that includes dementia care. I was fortunate enough to purchase it for my mom, and it assisted me greatly in being Mom's care leader. If you are not familiar with long-term care insurance, I will tell you a bit about it. Medical insurance, including Medicare, will not pay for hands-on care involving the activities of daily living. Most long-term insurance policies will pay for this hands-on care whether the care is in a facility or at home. It is good to have that choice, so look for policies that provide for both living arrangements. Make sure the one you are looking at includes dementia care. When a patient needs care for a very long time, it is usually due to dementia. Mom's policy covered care in both the home and a facility as well as covering dementia.

Purchasing long term care insurance for Mom is the best investment decision I have ever made in my life. I paid premiums for Mom's plan for 11 years before we needed to use the plan. Typically, you are allowed to stop paying premiums while you are getting benefit payments from the policy. We received payments from the policy for eight years for caregivers at home. We received more than five times more in benefits than we paid on premiums. Looking at it just financially, that is an amazing return on investment. More important, it gave me peace of mind that I had financial help in taking care of Mom. These payments made caring for Mom better and easier. When I needed 60-70 hours of care a week, the policy essentially covered all the hands-on care expenses. Later, when Mom needed around the clock care at home, the policy covered a little more than half the amount needed. This help was a lifesaver for me. It gave me great peace of mind.

I can't think of a more important investment than helping your loved one in this way. I have heard people tell me that long-term care insurance has changed recently. I recently purchased long-term care for both my sister and me. Things have not changed that much. There are still many long-term care plans available, and they work the same way they did when I purchased the coverage for Mom years ago. Premiums will go up some each year, but, as we know, so does everything else. Rates are regulated in most states, so the increases seem reasonable. It is important to know that your loved one will likely be asked to do a cognitive test to qualify for a plan that covers dementia. This is why it is very important to purchase the plan before your loved one starts showing symptoms of dementia. Please get ahead of the curve on this. You won't be sorry.

There are two basic types of long-term care insurance policies: traditional and hybrid. You can pay off both policies in a lump sum or make payments over time. There are still many wonderful carriers that offer both types of plans.

The traditional policy, which is what Mom had, is the kind that only reimburses you for your direct care expenses for activities of daily living. If you do not use the care, you do not receive anything from the insurance company. Most insurances like home or auto work this way. If you and your loved one are fortunate and don't need care, you lose the premiums you paid. Even if your loved one does not get Alzheimer's or another dementia, most people at some point will need some direct care, so it is a good option for many people. Hybrid policies, like traditional policies, provide direct caregiving expense reimbursement; however, with hybrids, if you don't use all or most of the reimbursement available for caregiving, the policy provides for a life insurance payment. Because the traditional policy does not provide a life insurance benefit, it will typically pay a little more for care (for the same premium) than the hybrid policy. Therefore, the traditional policy may be better for you if having a life insurance feature is not important to you or your loved one.

The earlier you purchase this important insurance the less expensive it will be, and because there is typically a cognitive test to qualify, purchase it early if you can. Dementia care needs are typically much longer in duration than other ailments and often require care around the clock. This is why these long-term care policies can be so important to Alzheimer's patients and their families. With people living longer, projections are that more than 30% of people over 65 will need dementia care in the not-too-distant future. A long-term care insurance policy will provide you with more options and peace of mind. Taking care of your loved one, especially at home, is a great experience when you have a great team helping and less financial worry. Because the breakthrough care pillars worked so well for Mom, she needed care for a very long time. Mom's long-term care policy gave me peace of mind that finances were not going to be an overwhelming barrier to having an exceptional care team.

If it is too late to buy long-term care insurance because your loved one already has dementia, families need to rally together to help. Don't be embarrassed to look to other family members for financial help. Also, these days most employers are more flexible helping employees take care of their family. Maybe rather than leaving your job altogether to be care leader, especially with other family members helping, maybe you could work part time, work remotely, or take a leave of absence during the time your loved needs the most care.

There may be other sources of financial help available. I know that if you deplete all your assets, Medicare can sometimes help with long-term care. In the resources section at the end of this book, you can find other sources to help you with this potential financial obstacle. Like my grandmother and my mom always said, "Where there is a will there is a way".

Overcoming the Time Obstacle

Being your loved one's care leader takes time. The needs of your loved one will be fewer in the early phases of dementia. This is the time to really learn about dementia and dementia care and start to build a superior care team. Investing your time early in finding a great care team that you trust can save you a great deal of time along the entire dementia journey.

Sometimes, family dynamics or geographic barriers won't allow you to get help from other family members. However, if you can get their help, they can assist you in overcoming many time challenges. Remember if you are the care leader you have ultimate accountability, but friends and family can assist you in providing care. There are many important potential roles for friends and family. They can help you research caregivers, agencies, or medical specialists. They can also help you by filling in with direct care and providing emotional support for you. Marina provided help for me in so many areas. She helped with direct care as well as gardening, cooking, laundry, and other important household tasks. Don't be afraid to ask for help. Asking for help is a sign of strength and not a weakness. You may be surprised how willing people are to help you; they will feel the grace of giving, positively transforming themselves during the journey, too.

There are many great tools and techniques that can help you with time pressures. None of these time tools is more powerful than the simple idea of prioritization. You will always have time for what is most important to you! First, reflect on what is truly important, and write these things down. The most important tasks are your A priorities. Taking care of Mom was always my A1 priority. I had B tasks and C tasks, but I put the most time on my A tasks. If you have B items and C items, you might try delegating those things to someone else. This will give you valuable time for your most important A priorities.

I am continually surprised at how powerful simple prioritization is. I learned and taught time management early in my career, and it has always helped me accomplish important goals in my career and my life overall. If you think time may be a barrier for you, there are time management resources at the end of the book.

Overcoming the Self Confidence Obstacle

How could I possibly have thought I could be Mom's care leader? I am not a medical expert or a caregiving expert. Sometimes, being an expert in a field can, paradoxically, prevent you from being as effective as you can be. Deep expertise can sometimes create biases and a closed mind to learning new ideas and finding frame breaking creative solutions to problems. For example, if I had already been an expert on caregiving, I might not have attempted to experiment and help Mom in so many different ways. I may not have tried so many small care improvements. I might have thought that since there was no "proven" research showing that a given aspect of care or nutritional element cured dementia, there was no use in trying. So, please shift your mindset from "lack of caregiving experience is a weakness" to thinking about it as a "strength." I wanted to learn from the experts and put various experts' ideas together in different and creative ways to try to make the biggest difference for Mom. What I lacked in experience in the beginning I made up for with passion, creativity, faith, and a curiosity and hunger to learn.

My hope is that your loved one's Alzheimer's journey will be healthy, long, and filled with as much happiness as possible. I know you will figure out what you need to know at each phase of their long journey. Feel the fear and do it anyway is one of the best pieces of advice I have ever been given. Look for your own biases and the mindsets that may be limiting you as you jump into this journey with your loved one. As you do more and try more care tactics, you will discover the confidence that comes with seeing how much better your loved one is doing. This confidence-experimentation-confidence cycle then becomes a continuous cycle of learning, trying, and improvement aimed at the mission of your loved one's longevity and joy. If you are afraid of being your loved one's active and accountable care leader, think about the fear your loved one has. Think about how afraid you would be if you are losing touch with who you are, not remembering loved ones, and feeling disoriented. Reflect on your loved one's tremendous fear and how your fear of being their care leader is small in comparison. Let their fear be a motivator for you to overcome your fear; let their need for you be a strength and a confidence builder for you.

If you encounter any of these obstacles or other potential obstacles to great care leadership for your loved one, take the actions necessary to break through that obstacle. You and your loved one will be glad you did. Remember what Winston Churchill said when faced with possible defeat during World War II: "Never, never, never, never give up!" Or, if you are not a history buff, listen to my grandmother who is speaking to us from heaven: "If it has been done before (and certainly if my grandson can do it), so can you!"

Chapter Summary

1. Passion to lead for your loved one, commitment to learning about dementia and dementia care, and being willing and able to build and motivate a championship care team comprise your leadership foundation for Breakthrough Care for your loved one. However, you still may encounter one or more of the potential care obstacles: 1) psychological, 2) financial, 3) time, or 4) self-confidence. Any of these perceived obstacles may rear its ugly head. To fully help your loved one, be ready to slay these obstacle beasts when they pop up.

2. *Psychological obstacle.* You may feel resentment for something your loved one has done in the past. Your loved one needs you now more than they ever have in the past. Try to tap into your love and your faith, to be the adult, and put any resentment to the side. Have faith that by helping your loved one in their biggest time of need, you are being the loving person your Maker has intended you to be. It may not be easy; seek help from a support group, an individual therapist, or friends. Remember, you are not alone; ask for help.

3. *Financial obstacle.* Leading the care for your loved one can be expensive. The amount of care your loved one needs, especially in the later phases of the disease, is extensive and may require 24/7 around-the-clock supervision and care. By far, the best thing you can do to help you help your loved one with this financially is to take out a long-term care insurance policy. It may seem expensive, but with dementia, the care needs are long-term and extensive. A long-term insurance plan, covering dementia, is likely to pay back many times over to help your loved one. However, if your loved one already has dementia, it may be too late as there is often cognitive testing to qualify. In that case, family members need to help each other. If your loved one needs financial help with care, ask other members of the

family to help financially, too. There is no shame in asking; your loved one needs you and the family. This is a devastating disease and if others in the family get dementia, they are likely to need help, too. Check the resources section for places to learn more about financial resources.

4. *Time obstacle.* When time is stretched too thin, it is often because we are not crystal clear on priorities. We either are not able to discern our true top priorities, or we spend too much time on lower priorities. You must decide what is most important to you; hopefully extending the life and joy of someone you love, who has a devastating disease, will pop into one of the highest priorities on your list. A first step is to take the time to reflect on what is truly important to you; what do you value the most? Time management resources in the resources section of the book will help you with tactics to be most efficient and align your time with your most important values and priorities.

5. *Self-confidence obstacle.* Know that no one can be a better care leader for your loved one than you. You have the passion and commitment to learn what you will need to know about being a great care leader. Being afraid to lead is very normal; you can break through all the obstacles to being a great care leader and truly help your loved one at the darkest and most difficult time in their lives.

The gift of being able to take care of your loved one while they are still alive is an incredible gift of love; it is the gift of life and the gift of joy. Please don't squander that gift with excuses or self-doubt. As you encounter perceived obstacles, work through the obstacle to reach the happiness on the other side. If you let one of these potential obstacles block you from being a wonderful care leader, you may regret this for the rest of your life. Choose to be empowered; please don't choose weakness or the victim rung of the Accountability Ladder. I know you will be a terrific, empowered care leader once you have made the commitment.

Breakthrough Pillar #1

Self-Care:

The Empowered Care Leader's Source of Renewable Energy

The first key to being an amazing care leader is leading the most important member of your care team …. you!! If you, as care leader, are not firing on all cylinders, Breakthrough Care won't go nearly as well. An energized and positively empowered care leader must lead your care team so that all these breakthrough care pillars are working at the needed exceptionally high level.

Check Your Mood Elevator

Before sharing what you can and should do to reenergize your leadership power, an important capability is knowing when you need reenergizing. There is a simple tool that can help immensely with this; it is called the Mood Elevator. The Mood Elevator was created by Larry Senn, a leading consultant, and author in the field of leadership to help leaders know when they have the needed positive energy or "mood" to be effective and when they don't. The higher buttons on the Mood Elevator are states that include being "grateful," "insightful," "creative," "resourceful," and "hopeful." If you do a gut or feeling check on yourself and have a sense you are in one of these higher mood states, you are high on the mood elevator and will be much more empowered and effective as a leader. However, if you do your feelings check and you feel "angry," "blaming," "depressed," or "stressed out," then you are lower on the Mood Elevator and won't be as effective. If you feel you are in one of these lower mood states, alarm bells should go off that you need to work to get renewed so that you can be in these higher, more effective mood states. Since you need to be a powerful care leader to help your loved one in breakthrough ways, please consider the following so you can stay high on the mood elevator. When you are up on the mood elevator, you will be both happier and more effective.

Passion: The Core of Renewable Energy

You must find the passion and motivation to lead for your loved one. It is critical when you are discouraged during the journey to be able to renew the energy to lead by tapping into the original drive that motivated you to help your loved one in the first place. This will encourage you to travel more easily over the bumps in the road on the dementia journey. This renewable energy source can come from many places. For me, it came from my deep love and respect for Mom and the faith Mom instilled in me. My higher purpose was to care for Mom. My leadership passion also came from my ancestors and the role models in my life. I saw them all demonstrating their love by gracefully and gladly making sacrifices for each other.

Your passion and renewable energy may come from similar sources or from totally different sources. No matter where the source of your drive to be your loved one's care leader comes from, know what it is, and call on it often. You may think things are too difficult. This is not the time to be discouraged; but it is a chance for you to tap into your passion and renew your loving care for your loved one who desperately needs you now. Being your loved one's care leader is a marathon and not a sprint. Your core passion to love and care for your loved one will become your renewable source of energy. Regularly remind yourself of how important taking care of your loved one is. Regularly check in with your higher purpose or our Maker to stay energized. The following are additional things to do to maintain the drive and positivity needed for the marathon.

Getting Caregiving Help for Renewal

Once again, you will very likely need and benefit from direct caregiving help. I opted not to have outside caregivers for the first four years of Mom's journey. As Mom entered the middle years of her Alzheimer's journey, I found myself staying up all night to watch her, dressing her, bathing her, serving her meals, and managing increasingly challenging medical care. Even with Marina's help it was too much. I felt exhausted and overwhelmed. Even though my passion and drive were sky high, I could feel my care effectiveness, energy, and capability dropping. I was not providing the care that Mom needed and deserved. This was the "aha" moment I needed to begin to find the best caregivers to help me. After much trial and error, I found and managed to keep an amazing small group of super talented caregivers. In Chapters 12-17, I will share how I found, led, retained, and motivated these incredible caregivers. I cannot begin to tell you how their loving help sustained and renewed my passion and drive for this incredible journey. I finally could get some sleep so I could be a better care leader. My wonderful team not only helped Mom immensely, but they also offered help, friendship, and support for me and my sister personally. Their wonderful talent and experience gave me good ideas and provided emotional and physical support. They became our trusted friends.

I also made many calls to the Alzheimer's Association hotline (800) 272-3900; I called to ask them how best to deal with Alzheimer's behavioral challenges, finding resources I needed, and to get a professional perspective on what was normal for each phase of Alzheimer's. Your local Alzheimer's Associations has many wonderful resources like seminars, hotlines, referrals, and support groups to help you on your care leader journey.

Talking with my caregivers, home-care agencies, and the Alzheimer's Association all renewed and reenergized me. Knowing that I was not alone in this journey gave me confidence. The support of others, confidence in what I was learning about Alzheimer's care, and the importance of my mission were all big energy renewal sources for me.

Emotional Help to Reframe and Recharge

It is very normal to experience a great amount of emotional angst and stress as you travel the Alzheimer's journey with your loved one. Seeing that person slowly slipping away is likely to be the most heart-wrenching experience in your life. I needed emotional support as well as direct care help. Mom declined mentally and physically at differing rates during her long journey. Some phases were much harder for me to experience than others. Fairly early on, Mom lost her speech. Losing the ability to talk with Mom was especially emotionally hard for me. Being so busy taking care of Mom in the early phase, I was at a big risk of internalizing all this anxiety. After my dad passed away, I had heart palpitations, dizziness, and other physical problems because I never verbalized my anxiety and grief. After I talked to a therapist, these medical issues subsided. I knew I did not want this to happen to me again, especially while caring for Mom, so I made sure that I had someone to talk to who could help me not internalize all this anxiety. There are studies that show that the stress of being a loved one's caregiver leads to caregivers getting medical problems. My therapist was a great sounding board for my feelings and offered some great ways to reframe what I was going through with Mom. I found therapy helped me with the grief of slowly losing Mom. If you do not have someone to talk to or a group to help you through this emotional journey, you risk missing many moments of joy during the journey. Another helpful idea is to join an Alzheimer's support group. There are many of these support groups in almost every community, and families are encouraged to join; they usually find much of the help they need there. The National Alzheimer's Association and its local chapters can help you find the right group.

This critical emotional renewal can come from a therapist, a support group, or other family members. It may even come from a very special soulmate friend or partner. Your loved one needs the best of you as care leader, so please get the emotional and physical help you need to run that marathon with your loved one.

Physical Activity and Social Connections for Renewed Energy

If, as care leader, you can create moments where you can connect with friends and stay physically active, you will be recharged and positive. Your loved one with dementia will benefit from your positive attitude. When I had moments of time I would prioritize going for short walks in the neighborhood. I would also try to make at least some kind of social connection at least a couple of times a week even if only for brief periods of time. My friends were a great support and patiently listened to me talk about my caregiving challenges. At times, I just needed a distraction from caregiving that my friends provided. You may have very limited time as care leader, but physical activity and social connections are very important to maintaining your energy and positivity. I would always take my phone with me during these recharge breaks. My caregivers were very talented, and they knew my brief time away was important for me. I cannot remember a single time when I was called back because there was a caregiving problem or emergency. Because I hired the best, I trusted my family of superstar caregivers; Mom was in good hands, and so was I.

Faith, Hope, and Love as Recharger

I found myself saying a lot of short prayers for Mom, for my wonderful caregivers, for my sister, and for my own strength, tenacity, and capability to help Mom through our Alzheimer's journey. I am so grateful that Mom raised me in faith; this helped me tap into the faith I needed during this time. I hope that you, too, can tap into your faith to help you and your loved one during their journey. Even though Mom had lost her words, I know that her faith carried her through her Alzheimer's journey, too. Luisa, one of our five remarkable long-term caregivers would occasionally pray with Mom. Even though Mom could not say a word, I saw Mom smile as a loving glow came over her when Luisa prayed with her.

When I saw these moments of joy radiate from Mom, my strength would be renewed, too. I knew even when Mom lost some cognitive ability or physical ability and changed emotionally, her soul was always there and would always be there. These holy moments of joy were critical in giving me new energy to learn more and do more for Mom's care. Being in gratitude gave me positive energy. I tried to stay grateful for Mom, my family, my care team, my life, and my friends.

Through the tough dementia care marathon, you will need to find your own sources of powerful renewable energy that work best for you! To be your best, these renewable energy sources are very important to keep you positive and empowered; you are the foundation as care leader for your loved one living longer and happier. If the foundation is weak, not much breakthrough happens.

Summary

1. Your energy, drive, and positivity to take care of your loved one at the highest level is important for bringing the necessary excellence to the breakthrough care pillars. You and your positive energy and leadership become the game changer for your loved one.

2. It will be very hard to sustain your energy for the care leader marathon without renewable sources of energy.

   a) Tap into the *internal sources* of renewal like your core passion and your faith to help your loved one. You must find it and come back to tap into it when you are tired, scared, or discouraged. Focus on the positive, and try to stay grateful and high on the mood elevator. If you believe in a higher power, pray. All these *internal sources* of energy and renewal can help strengthen your resolve.

   b) *External sources* of energy renewal are also very important, too. These include:

   a. care help from great caregiver agencies and Alzheimer's associations;

   b. emotional support from therapists and formal Alzheimer's support groups—you can find these support groups through your local Alzheimer's Associations, your church/synagogue, or online;

   c. Social connections, which are vital for renewal—connecting with friends and family to feel supported, take a break from caregiving, and have a little needed fun; and

   d. physical exercise, which is important for energy and your health—walking or other forms of exercise to feel energized and have a little necessary fun.

Breakthrough Pillar #2
Safety is the Gateway to Happiness, Health, and Longevity

Why do I start with safety, and why is great safety a game changer? Safety does not seem like a breakthrough pillar. It sounds too basic, right? But consider: dementia patients are more prone to falling, choking, pneumonia, sepsis, and other secondary medical issues which often prevent them from living longer and happier. Many of these secondary medical conditions can be avoided with excellent safety practices. If Mom had not been safe, it is highly unlikely that she would have lived as long or as happily as she did.

Hospital stays almost always are a setback for an Alzheimer's patient. Most Alzheimer's patients get confused with unfamiliar surroundings, including unknown staff members, in a hospital. The nutrition, exercise, stimulation, and other breakthrough pillars that you may have worked so hard to establish are often impossible to maintain during and after a hospital stay. In hospitals, surgery, anesthesia, pain pills, tranquilizers, and sleeping pills (often given) will reduce the cognitive reserve that you have been preciously trying to hold onto for your loved one. Cognitive reserve is our reserved brain power. When someone has Alzheimer's or another dementia, their normal brainpower is very limited. As a result, drawing down this already very limited cognitive reserve can cause a big mental decline. There is nothing good about a hospital visit for a dementia patient. Good safety really can help keep your loved one out of the hospital.

Even if an accident or illness does not send your loved one to a hospital, it can significantly reduce mobility. Mobility is key for a dementia patient's physical, mental, and emotional health. If a fall or other avoidable medical condition leaves your loved one sedentary, without the ability to exercise or move properly, it is usually a big setback. Movement enhances physical health, cognition, fun, and positivity. You can't be out and have fun or do much of anything if you are confined to a bed recovering from a fall or other medical problem.

There is a concept I learned working in human resources that helped me think about safety for Mom. The concept is borrowed from retail consulting; the thought is understanding "customer experience touchpoints." I learned about this while co-leading a new restaurant experience design project. It came from Lou Carbone, a terrific retail customer experience expert. If you walk into a store, put yourself into the mind of a customer, and ask, "What does the customer experience at every point in their experience?" From the moment customers approach the store until after they leave, and even later, what do they see? What do they hear? What are they likely to sense, think, and feel? Are customers' experiences what you want them to have at each "touchpoint." Similarly, your loved will have daily and weekly experiences. At every moment or point, your loved one will have safety, cognitive, and emotional encounters (touchpoints). They will have thoughts and feelings about what they see, touch, and hear at every moment in their day. For every movement and encounter they have, they can be either safer or less safe at that moment. Like a retailer who might think ahead and design every customer experience touchpoint, I tried to think about and anticipate everything Mom encountered in her daily routine as a touchpoint for her. Each experience related either to her safety and health, her cognitive and physical stimulation, or her emotions and happiness. In Chapters 23 and 24, I will share what I did to design experience touchpoints for Mom to enhance her cognition, fun, movement, love, and familiarity. However, safety comes first; without safety, not much else might matter.

The following safety touchpoints (encounters with the physical environment) are important for a care leader to anticipate, being sure to minimize or eliminate risk. If I did not anticipate and eliminate safety risks, Mom would be in danger. When your loved one's safety is at risk, breakthrough becomes irrelevant. All it takes is one safety lapse to have a major problem and major setback for your loved one.

If your loved one is in a facility, it is essential to observe each of these safety touchpoints, too. Check the facility at different times and on different days, and be sure each of the following safety solutions are in place for each risk below. If they are not all in place, try to influence the facility manager to update their safety protocols and ensure excellent execution. If they don't upgrade their safety, consider moving your loved one to a safer place.

CHAPTER 6

Preventing a Tragic Fall

There are several things about dementia patients that pose safety challenges. The first major safety priority is making sure your loved one doesn't fall. Falling can lead to brain injury, broken bones, or sprains that limit mobility or worse for your loved one. Because the brain and body often don't cooperate in a dementia patient, muscles can tighten up resulting in your loved one shuffling their legs and feet. When your loved one's feet shuffle under them, they can easily trip and fall. This shuffling safety risk is extra risky when your loved one changes direction or when starting to walk from a sitting or lying down position. Alzheimer's patients can also be prone to being easily agitated. Someone who is suddenly agitated or confused can lose focus and momentarily forget how to walk safely.

First, make sure your loved one only wears good sturdy walking shoes with tie laces. Mom always loved her Easy Spirit walking shoes and owned them in a few different colors. She walked with more confidence and stability in these tie shoes. If your loved one has a hard time tying their shoes, you can tie them or have your caregiver tie the laces. Walking shoes with tie laces are more stable than other types of shoes.

Second, a simple walker is also a good tool to reduce fall risk. I strongly encourage the use of a walker. A simple sturdy walker is inexpensive and covered by most insurances. I think some people believe that a walker implies that a person is crippled or handicapped. You or your loved one may not like that inference. That is not the way to think about it; rather, a walker is insurance. A walker is a basic safety tool for anyone who has any shuffle or struggle walking. I have been told that some people don't think their loved one would want to use a walker. They believe their loved one's need for independence would make them not like to use a walker. I mistakenly thought that was true for Mom, too, but we figured out that if we made the walker a positive, fun experience instead of a sterile, medical, or losing your independence thing, Mom gladly used the walker. With the Breakthrough Care underlying principle of "always make it fun," we hung Mom's favorite stuffed animals, little bangles, and her Betty Boop key chain (Mom loved Betty Boop) on the walker. Mom suddenly wanted to use her walker because we made it fun and positive for her. Also, I know Mom loved and trusted us and knew that we were looking out for her safety and enjoyment. Because Mom lost her speech so early in her journey, I did not know for sure, but I had the feeling she also did things we wanted her to do, like using the walker, because she also wanted to make us happy. This contributed to Mom being as cooperative as she was.

Mom was able to use the walker to walk around the house throughout her Alzheimer's journey. Outside, in new surroundings, there was less risk if she used her wheelchair. With a walker, people might accidentally bump her or there might be unusual stairs, uneven sidewalks, and other things that could cause her to lose her balance and fall. The number one thing was to avoid a fall that could send Mom to the hospital or worse. Mom may have lost a small amount of opportunity for exercise or a little sense of independence by using her wheelchair for our daily outings, but that was worth the big gain in eliminating the fall risk.

Mom loved going out each day. She had so much joy and had a big smile when she saw new and familiar sites and people, especially children, during our daily outings. Going out was the highlight of her day. After Mom went on our daily outing, she was calmer and happier at home. Taking Mom out every day was a pleasure because she experienced so much joy, and I knew she was safe with the wheelchair. With Mom's wheelchair, we could also cover more ground, too; we could go to the park, to Sprinkles for her children's scoop of ice cream, shopping, and other places she loved. Mom's wheelchair was a "travel wheelchair," not one of those bigger wider ones you usually see. Travel wheelchairs are safe but much narrower and lighter. These wheelchairs are easy to take in and out of the trunk, and because they are narrower, they are also easier than a regular wheelchair to navigate through the narrow aisles of many stores.

As with Mom's walker, we decorated Mom's wheelchair with all the fun things Mom loved. Many people on our outings would comment on how "fun and happy" the decorations looked on Mom's wheelchair, and she would smile really big when she heard these comments. She especially enjoyed children approaching her and saying they liked something on her wheelchair. Mom loved children. Going out every day brought so much happiness for Mom.

I have been told by families that they are concerned about going out with their loved one with a walker or wheelchair because there are stairs involved in getting to the car. Yes, stairs are difficult if using a walker or wheelchair. At our home, there is only one step for Mom to go over with her walker on the way to the car. We were able to help Mom over that step with her walker. However, if your loved one's home has a couple of steps, there are now portable ramps you could lay down. I only used it occasionally, but I bought one of these portable ramps on Amazon. They are light, very sturdy, and not expensive; they have a rough surface so your loved one won't slip. They are foldable so you make them a little longer or shorter and store them in your car. I don't recommend them for a staircase but just to go over a couple of steps they work very well.

I have also heard families say they don't like taking their loved one out because they worry about them being agitated in public; some families feel a little embarrassed by their loved one's agitated behavior. Alzheimer's patients thrive on routine and what is safe and familiar. If you safely take your loved one out on a familiar route with the same helpers and make the outing fun, your loved one will likely feel very secure and comforted. This will help them be calmer and happier and less agitated. If your loved one still happens to get agitated, correction does not help. Rather, reframe the situation into a positive one. People around you will be surprisingly understanding of a dementia person who is agitated. Rather than being embarrassed by your loved one in public, reframe the situation, and be proud that you are taking them out and helping in a fun and special way. Everyone you may meet is also thinking that you are terrific to take such good care of your loved one. They are thinking that you should be proud of yourself (and they would be right).

Staying mobile, especially when going out to fun places, is great for your loved one's outlook, their physical and mental stimulation, and their fun and happiness. If they are safe, there is nothing better or more empowering for them, and for you, than to take your loved one out each day for a wonderful and enjoyable daily adventure.

Chapter Summary

1. Have good walking shoes with tie laces.

2. Use a walker if your loved one is shuffling, wobbly, or not sure-footed. Consider decorating the walker with what your loved one likes to make it fun, especially if there is any resistance to using it.

3. Use a wheelchair when outside (or if needed in general) if there is any walking difficulty or hesitation. You can also, like the walker, make the wheelchair fun by decorating it with fun things your loved one might like.

4. Throw away all throw rugs (they are called "throw rugs") and be sure flooring is not hard or slippery.

CHAPTER 7

Bathroom Safety

You want your loved one to stay mobile for as long as possible. Regardless of whether your loved one's dementia has progressed to the point where they need assistance in the bathroom or not, the following safety elements will reduce the risk for all the bathroom safety touchpoints.

First, most bathrooms have tile floors. Tile is hard and very slippery when it's wet. Since water is often spilled on bathroom tiles, the bathroom is a very dangerous place for your loved one with dementia. Many of the safety products come from learning from children's safety. Children's playrooms often have rubber tile squares that are a jigsaw. They fit together and can cover many areas where your loved one could fall. They are textured and have thick rubber which reduces the risk of slipping and are much softer in case there is an accidental fall.

I used these simple rubber jigsaw tiles in Mom's bathroom from the very beginning to reduce the impact of a fall. When you search on Amazon or Google, these are called rubber playmats or play tiles. Many retailers carry them. These play tiles come in many sizes and fun colors. You can put them all over the bathroom floor for less than the cost of dinner out.

The second bathroom safety suggestion is to make sure you have an "over the toilet" chair. These devices go over the regular toilet, raise up the toilet seat a little, and have rails to hold onto that help your loved one stand up more easily and safely. Getting up from a low toilet without rails to help you push up is very difficult and risky. These over-toilet chairs make toileting much safer. They are more comfortable and very sturdy, and they cost less than a breakfast out. Being a little higher also reduces constipation a bit, too. One of the convenient things about these chairs is that they can be easily transported. You can install them yourself by simply placing them over the toilet. Mom was so much more comfortable and secure getting on and off the toilet with one of these over- toilet chairs.

Third, if your toilet is near a wall, it is a good idea to attach a safety handrail on the wall next to the toilet. Your loved one can hold onto the safety rail when they change direction or go from sitting to standing in the bathroom. Later, when your loved one needs help bathing, dressing, or toileting, they can hold onto this handrail while being dressed or cleaned. Get handrails that are screwed into the wall rather than the ones that attach with a suction cup. I tried the suction cup kind, and they are not safe; they come off the wall too easily. If you are not handy (like me), a handyman can attach the bathroom handrails. Neither the rail nor the installation is expensive, and it may add to the value of your home as well as give you great peace of mind knowing that you have improved another safety touchpoint and made your loved one a little safer.

The next major bathroom fall risk touchpoint occurs when bathing. If your loved one is still mobile, a walk-in shower is much safer than a tub. With some help, Mom could step over the small step into the stand-up shower for almost all her Alzheimer's journey. A traditional bathtub is far too hard for most seniors and especially for dementia patients to step into.

Standing in a slippery shower is not a good idea for any senior. We used a plastic shower chair for Mom to sit on while showering. These portable shower chairs have rubber feet, handrails, and are very sturdy. They are comfortable, safe, and inexpensive. Shower chairs are readily available on Amazon and in local hospital supply stores. Sitting while showering really does reduce the fall risk significantly.

Another important safety tool in the bathroom for a more comfortable shower experience is a handheld shower wand. With a handheld shower wand, your loved one can comfortably and safely sit on the shower chair. With the hand-held shower wand, there is a long very light flexible metal or plastic hose your loved one can use to clean themselves or be cleaned by the caregiver. The water can be aimed more precisely without splashing everywhere. This allows the caregiver to step into the shower to help without getting wet. The precise water aiming also helped Mom get cleaner, and she was less agitated because the water was focused and not splashing over her face and everywhere else. Mom enjoyed her showers, felt safe, and had fun in the shower with her caregivers. These hand-held shower wands are available for only a few dollars at any hardware store or big box retailer. I could even attach it myself (and you already know I'm not handy).

Water that is too hot or too cold could also be problematic. If your loved one is still able to shower with little or no help, they may not be able to adjust the correct shower temperature to a safe and comfortable temperature. If this is the case, there are devices available to auto-adjust the water temperature The caregiver can also easily adjust the temperature to the safest water temperature.

However, during the very late phase of Mom's Alzheimer's journey, even a sit-down chair shower with a hand wand was difficult for her. We would skip the sit-down shower and instead opt for a sponge bath. We would sometimes give Mom a sponge bath after she went to the bathroom because she was already safely seated on the raised toilet seat. We would simply use a washcloth and a basin to wash her and put a big warm towel around her for drying off. We used a spray bottle to wet her hair and used a gentle shampoo on her scalp. Occasionally we would use dry shampoo if it looked like Mom was a little fussy that day and might not want to get her head wet.

In a facility, these bathroom safety touchpoints are also very important. The bathroom is the most dangerous room in the house or facility for your loved one. The hard tile and slippery floor and metal fixtures can cause a severe injury if there is a fall. Many Alzheimer's patients living in a facility have fallen and suffered terrible injuries in the bathroom. Periodically, it is a good idea to observe your loved one's caregivers to make sure these safety pillars are in place and used for every single trip your loved one takes to the bathroom. In this chapter summary, I list all the safety equipment and tools that you and your loved one's caregivers needs ensure safety overall.

Chapter Summary

1. Put rubber kids' tiles over hardwood or tile floor.

2. Use an over-toilet chair with rails to raise toilet seat and help them get up.

3. Install permanent handrails near the toilet and in the shower.

4. Don't use a traditional tub; it is too much of a risk for your loved one to step over the side safely. Use a low step-in shower instead.

5. Use a sturdy rubber footed shower chair in the shower.

6. Replace the regular shower head with a handheld shower wand.

Bedroom Safety

Just like you don't want the bathroom floor to be hard, it also isn't a good idea for the bedroom floor to be hard or of a material that is slippery and can cause a fall. Ideally, a carpeted bedroom is best so long as the carpet isn't shaggy or too thick. If there are throw rugs, towels, or anything slippery or bumpy in the bedroom or hallway, take them out. Throw rugs are a major fall risk for a shuffling senior. If the bedroom is a hardwood floor or other hard materials, you don't have to change the entire flooring but rather you can put the same rubber jigsaw tiles down that you used in the bathroom. In our case, my mom's bedroom already had short pile carpeting. Many facilities have hard linoleum or composite floors which I know are easier to clean but are not as safe as soft pile carpeting. If your loved one needs to be in a facility, please make sure you choose a facility where there is short pile carpet or other very soft flooring especially in the bedroom and walkways.

Second, after soft safe flooring, I encourage you to be sure there is a bedrail on your loved one's bed—if not on both sides, then at least on the side of the bed where your loved one turns while sleeping. Bedrails are important so that your loved one does not accidentally roll off the bed. Also, if they need assistance to go to the bathroom, they are prevented from getting up too quickly on their own and risking a fall. There are many kinds of bedrails that I looked at for Mom. The one I liked the best were the "half rails." They are about 3½' long and about a foot high. When Mom was lying down, they measured from about Mom's shoulder to her thigh. I like these because they stopped Mom from accidentally rolling out of bed or falling if she tried to go to the bathroom without a caregiver helping her but also made it easy to get her in and out of bed.

The bed's half rails were very safe and looked nice in her room. The long full-length bedrails, like most hospital bedrails, may look and be too confining for your loved one while providing negligible additional safety. As with Mom's walker, we decorated her bedrails with her favorite dolls, favorite-colored afghans, and stuffed animals to make her room fun and warm. This supported our breakthrough principle of making every touchpoint, even the bedrails, fun, comforting, and familiar. The bedrails, like magic, went from clinical to fun. In addition to giving the bedrail a warm nice look, the afghan and blankets on the bedrail protected Mom from accidentally scraping her skin on the metal. As Mom got older, her skin became very thin and easily torn or bruised—and prone to a skin infection—if she bumped the bedrail. These bedrails are inexpensive on Amazon or at a hospital supply store and are very easy to set up. They are portable; the straps that hold them go under the mattress. They are quite stable and secure. When lying down, your loved one won't feel any securing rods or bumps under the mattress.

The third bedroom safety item needed is a motion alarm or two. There are many kinds of alarms you can use in your loved one's bedroom. The one that I found to be the best for Mom was a small motion-activated sensor alarm. The sensors are small and can be placed on the bedroom rug or chair. They measure only two inches high and an inch wide. If your loved one starts to get out of bed or out of a chair, the visual sensor is triggered, and the small handheld receiver alarm will go off. The range of most of these motion alarms is the size of most homes. If you must step away from your loved one to do something in another room, you can still hear the motion alarm go off if your loved one starts to get up. You can run in and make sure your loved one is safe. I had two of these sensors on the floor in Mom's bedroom. The sensors are easy to operate and are battery powered. You just put them in the field of motion you want to monitor and turn them on. You can take the small receiver anywhere in the house, and you will know if your loved one is about to get up. By doing this I made the home much safer for Mom. Mom did not wander around the house or try to get out of the house like some Alzheimer's patients do. If your loved tends to wander, you can put the motion sensor alarms in places that would signal to you that your loved one is on the move.

Some facilities and many hospitals use bed alarms if they think a patient might have a fall. These alarms usually attach to the mattress so if the patient gets up, the weight of their body is no longer on the mattress, triggering the alarm. I looked at this kind for Mom but didn't like them as much as the motion sensor alarms. Motion sensors were better for Mom because if Mom's legs were over the side of the bed for some reason, the alarm would sound, and the caregiver could come in quickly to help her. If I used a bed alarm, Mom would have to be standing on the floor before the alarm would sound. Once your loved one is standing, there is already a fall risk. The extra few seconds difference between it going off when her feet were over the bed versus her already standing could be the difference between falling and not falling. Another big advantage is that the motion alarms are portable and can be put anywhere you are worried your loved one may go. I insisted Mom be watched all the time; if you put a motion sensor alarm next to the chair your loved one likes, you can tell when they start to get up. You can also turn the alarm off from the receiver as you enter the room so your loved one will not be disturbed by the alarm going off when you enter the room. I purchased both these amazing little motion alarms for less than $50 on Amazon.

Finally, learning from children again, I found these rubber furniture edge guards that I put on any sharp edges on furniture in the bedroom and in other rooms in the house. These were so great because Mom had such fragile skin that any bump or tear on a sharp furniture edge could cause a bigger problem like a bruise or infection. Also, if your loved one falls against or on a piece of the furniture's sharp edge, they can really get hurt by a sharp edge.

Chapter Summary

1. Don't have hard flooring in the bedroom. If there is no short carpet in the bedroom, use rubber kids tiles on the floor. Never use throw rugs in the bedroom or walking areas of the home.

2. Put portable motion alarm sensors on the carpet floor near the bed.

3. Put safety bedrails (half rails) on the bed.

4. Put on rubber edge guards, especially on the bedroom furniture.

CHAPTER 9

Kitchen and Meal Safety

Because Alzheimer's patients later in their dementia don't always recognize the risk of something, it is important for you to anticipate and be careful to protect them from sharp objects, chemicals, or corrosive materials that are often found around the kitchen. Learning from childcare again, we put child locks on most reachable cabinets and cupboards.

Second, the stove is another area where your loved one can get hurt. Many Alzheimer's patients may lose their memory of a stove being hot. If this is the case, keep an eye on them in the kitchen and cover your cooking surfaces with something like a pot top or covering when you are not in the kitchen. Many dementia patients may still know that the stove is hot but may forget to turn the stove off. If this is the case, there are devices you can put on the stove to automatically turn the stove off at a certain time in case your loved has forgotten to turn the stove off.

Third, eating is another area that could be risky for your loved one with Alzheimer's or dementia. As their dementia progresses, your loved one may have trouble remembering to chew their food well or may have trouble swallowing their food properly. A couple of tips really helped me with these potential problems. First, I learned that child utensils, small firm rubber spoons and forks, were better for Mom than regular utensils. When Mom started having trouble chewing and swallowing well, a smaller amount fit on the child's fork or spoon and made the possibility of her choking on food less of a risk. Also, like many dementia patients far along in their journey, Mom, like a very young child, liked to bite down on things. So, another big advantage of these rubber child utensils was that if Mom would bite down on a rubber spoon or fork, it was virtually impossible for her to hurt her mouth or teeth. I found these child utensils at Walmart, but they can be found in most children's food supply aisles in many markets.

As Mom's chewing and swallowing risk worsened, it was important to monitor the speed of Mom's swallowing. Mom fed herself throughout her journey, but we would watch her to be sure she swallowed before she took another bite. Mom really looked forward to eating, and we wanted her to be as independent as possible and to be able to feed herself as she enjoyed her meals. Watching Mom swallow was easy to do by simply watching her throat move when she swallowed any food. As we managed the speed at which she ate, she got the hang of the rhythm of swallowing before taking in more food. In the beginning, Mom resisted us managing the speed at which she ate, but soon she became more comfortable and learned the rhythm of proper swallowing before she took more food.

What Mom ate was also important because swallowing is such a problem for dementia patients. We would make sure Mom's food was cut into small bites and that her vitamins and prescription pills were small enough for her to swallow. If the pills were too large, we would cut them, crush them, or purchase them in a liquid form. This was surprisingly easy to do and much safer than expecting Mom to swallow the kind of giant horse pills that exist for some prescriptions and vitamins. Very late in Mom's Alzheimer's journey, it was suggested that a thickening agent be used to create a thicker density in the liquids that she drank like soups or juice. The thickening agent, which is easy to add to drinks and soups, makes swallowing much safer because it avoids material getting into the lungs and developing aspiration pneumonia. You can find many over-the-counter thickeners for this purpose that are easy to use.

Mom would eat on her own while her caregiver watched to be sure she was safe. Although eating safely is very serious for Alzheimer's patients, Mom's caregivers made it fun, too. If Mom was eating too fast, they would tease her and have fun with it rather than being critical. Mom would smile at the teasing. They also, if Mom was eating too fast, might take a brief distraction break to show Mom a magazine photo she liked. Mom really enjoyed eating and because we anticipated these eating risk touchpoints, we avoided any choking and related problems with Mom.

Chapter Summary

1. Remove dangerous chemicals and sharp objects from the kitchen.

2. Put children's safety locks on the cabinets.

3. Consider using children's size rubber utensils to limit food size and reduce biting metal and hurting teeth or mouth.

4. Chop, dice, cut finely, or liquify food to reduce swallowing risk. Make sure your loved one swallows (watch their throat move) before eating more food.

CHAPTER 10

COVID, Viruses, and Germ Safety

Finally, I would like to talk about COVID and Virus Safety for your loved one. My mom was in her late stage of Alzheimer's during the beginning of the COVID epidemic. When anyone came into the house, I made sure they were masked, gloved, recently tested, and did not have any symptoms of COVID. For our ongoing caregivers, I made sure they were COVID safe. That meant they had to be COVID tested and not exposed to any other person who hadn't been recently tested. For viruses overall, it helped that I was able to give our small group of caregivers enough working hours that they did not have to pick up any hours at another workplace, where they might contract a virus and spread it to Mom.

I used High-Efficiency Particulate Air (HEPA) filter machines in each of the rooms even before Mom's Alzheimer's. I have bad allergies, and these HEPA filters help me. They were an added benefit to help Mom avoid some viruses and germs. Virus safety is critical even if there is no pandemic. Colds, flus, viral pneumonia, shingles, c-diff, and other transmitted diseases can be devastating to the elderly and especially to elderly dementia patients. In a facility or community, there are so many different caregivers, patients, and other staff and visitors who step in and out of patients' rooms. That is why, in my opinion, following these safety protocols is especially important. It is so much easier to manage who comes in and out of your home, which may be safer than having your loved one exposed to many different people with various viruses in a community setting.

Chapter Summary

1. If there is a pandemic or any other significant virus risk, ask all who encounter your loved one to get tested and mask up.

2. Use high quality HEPA Filter machines in every room your loved goes in.

3. Minimize, where possible, group contact or large gatherings with your loved one.

4. If you need your loved one to wear a mask, dementia patients often pull their mask off; if this is the case, make sure others are wearing one in the presence of your loved one, especially during flu season and other high virus risk times.

CHAPTER 11

Safety Summary & Overall Safety Equipment List

All the above safety precautions were key for me as care leader to make sure all Mom's safety touchpoints were completely safe. The peace of mind knowing Mom was as safe as I could make her was well worth a few hundred dollars to get the right safety equipment and tools for the house. I encourage you to think about safety as a series of physical touchpoints that your loved one may encounter in their routine for each hour, day, and week. The key is to anticipate each risk touchpoint, then make the change to make it a little safer.

If Mom had been in a facility or community, I would have made sure all these safety measures were in place there, too. Safety is the foundation of all great breakthrough care for your loved one. Falling, choking, and aspiration pneumonia (coming from not swallowing well) are the biggest causes of a shortened life for both Alzheimer's patients and the elderly in general.

My paternal grandmother, who lived in a facility in New York, was in her 90s and didn't have dementia. However, she fell in the care facility's bathroom and died very quickly after her fall. I have heard from many people who have had the same horror stories about their loved one who suffered tremendously from a fall or other safety problem. Safety is extremely important for any older person, and the dangers are largely preventable

Safety is the most important factor in extending the life and the happiness of your loved one. This is true whether you are leading safety for your loved one at home or monitoring the safety of the facility. For me, safety at home was easier to do than I originally thought. Having a safety checklist, like the one below, could be part of your facility selection criteria. If after close observations, you find your loved one's place of living does not receive an A+ from you, the Safety Commissioner, please find a new home for your loved one. If you opt for care at home, use this safety checklist to make these small adjustments in your home to achieve a big improvement in safety for your loved one. At the end of the book there are additional resources for learning more about safety. In Chapters 15 & 16, when I discuss leading caregivers, I will revisit how to help caregivers manage safety.

Overall Safety Equipment List

The following is a list of the tools and equipment from these Safety Chapters.

Overall Fall Prevention

1. Have good walking shoes with tie laces.

2. Use a walker if your loved one is shuffling, wobbly, or not sure-footed. Consider decorating the walker with what your loved one likes to make it fun, especially if there is any resistance to using it.

3. Use a wheelchair when outside (or if needed in general) if there is any walking difficulty or hesitation. You can also, like the walker, make the wheelchair fun by decorating it with fun things your loved one might like.

4. Remove all throw rugs, and be sure flooring is not hard or slippery.

Bathroom Safety

1. Put rubber kids' tiles over hard or hard tile floor.

2. Use an over-toilet chair with rails to raise the toilet seat and help users get up.

3. Install permanent handrails near the toilet and in the shower.

4. Don't use a traditional tub; it is too much of a risk to step over the side safely. Use a low step-in shower instead.

5. Use a sturdy rubber-footed shower chair in the shower.

6. Replace the regular shower head with a handheld shower wand.

Bedroom Safety

1. Don't have hard flooring in the bedroom. If there is no short carpet in the bedroom, use kids' rubber tiles on the floor. Never use throw rugs in the bedroom or walking areas of the home.

2. Put portable motion alarm sensors on the soft floor or carpet near the bed.

3. Put safety bedrails on the bed.

4. Put on rubber edge guards, especially on the bedroom furniture.

Kitchen and Meal Safety

1. Remove dangerous chemicals and sharp objects from the kitchen.

2. Put children's safety locks on the cabinets.

3. Consider using children's size rubber utensils to limit food size and reduce biting risk.

4. Chop, dice, cut finely, or liquify food to reduce swallowing risk. Make sure your loved one swallows (watch their throat move) before eating more food.

Covid/Virus/Germ Safety

1. If there is a pandemic or any other significant virus risk, ask all who will encounter your loved one to get tested and/or mask up.

2. Use high quality HEPA filter machines in any room your loved goes in.

3. Minimize, where possible, group contact or large gatherings with your loved one.

4. If you need your loved one to wear a mask, keep in mind that dementia patients often pull their mask off; if this is the case, make sure others are wearing one in the presence of your loved one, especially during flu season and other high virus risk times.

Breakthrough Pillar #3

Build the Finest

Care Team Ever

Your loved one's happiness and longevity have everything to do with the care team with which you surround them. Your loved one's care team provides safety, medical care, mobility, cognitive and physical stimulation, fun, comfort, reassurance, and love. Your care team is your loved one's entire world. There is nothing more important than surrounding your loved one with the finest care team you can find. Your exemplary care team will be comprised of caregivers, doctors, other medical specialists (e.g., physical therapists, podiatrists, dentists), and other important helpers (hair cutters, etc.).

As a former HR leader, I learned that the best way to think about assembling the best team is to be clear about what you are looking for. Like an archer, you must know where the target is. I always found it useful to think about this in two categories: first, there are baseline skills or skills you must possess just to be considered for the team, and second, there are differentiating skills or skills that make you stand out from the crowd and make you excellent. The baseline skills are a must, but the differentiating skills are the difference between a good team member and a truly incredible team member. We want only truly incredible team members to take care of our loved ones. It is in assembling a truly incredible care team that the magic of breakthrough care and breakthrough results will happen. Competence and experience with dementia are the baseline for direct caregivers and medical specialists. If they don't have these basics, they should not even be considered for your team. So, what are the differentiators? What are these magic skills that if everyone on your team has will bring breakthrough results for your loved one? The magic will come from their level of compassion, creativity, and sensory intelligence.

Compassion, Creativity, and Sensory Intelligence

Compassion, creativity, and sensory intelligence, built on the strong foundation of experience and technical competence, is at the core of anyone who is truly going to help your loved one in these remarkable ways. The good news is that these three skills are usually found in the same people. Jenn Granneman and Andre Solo (2024), in a wonderful book called *Sensitive* found in their studies that people with high compassion and empathy often are the most creative and the most tuned into noticing and observing their environment (sensory intelligence). So why are these three skills so important for your loved one, and how are they linked together?

Compassion & Empathy. Having every member of your team, and especially your direct caregivers, be highly compassionate and empathetic brings patience, connection, warmth, and love to your loved one. Highly empathetic people are better listeners and will be tuned into what your loved one is feeling and what they need and want. As dementia patients lose their ability to speak, a highly empathetic and compassionate care team member will take the time to know your loved one and will sense, with their feeling and intuition, what they need or want. I saw this with my highly empathetic care team members as Mom completely lost her speech. Highly empathetic and compassionate people are also usually more curious about others; they will get to know your loved one and because they care deeply about others' feelings, they will want to and will creatively make your loved one happy, secure, and comforted.

You also want your care team's physicians and other specialists to be experienced with dementia and technically strong, but you also want them to be highly compassionate, empathetic, and creative too. Not only will they treat your loved one better when they interact with them but because empathetic people are better listeners and care more about others, your empathetic medical team will listen better and be more tuned into your loved one's needs and symptoms and take more time with them. All this listening and empathy will lead to a more comprehensive diagnosis of their needs resulting in much better care.

Creativity. Creativity is also very important for every member of your care team. You will want your loved one's direct caregivers to use their creativity to come up with creative and fun games and other creative activities to help your loved one have more cognitive and physical stimulation, fun, and comfort. Your creative caregivers will also bring more creativity and artistry to how they deal with any agitation or resistance your loved one may have. The caregiver's creativity and empathy will come together here to creatively redirect or use creative loving humor with your loved one when they are agitated. This will leave your loved one much happier than if your caregiver was frustrated, critical, or adamant.

You also want your medical care team to be creative. Creative people are better at seeing connections between things that create better solutions. A creative physician will be better at seeing connections between symptoms to form a better diagnosis of your loved one's condition. A creative medical specialist will also be better at combining therapies in new ways leading to better medical outcomes for your loved one. Later, I share how two of Mom's "medical gurus" creatively mixed therapies to cure Mom of a chronic medical condition that the other good (but less creative) physician specialists could not cure.

Why are highly empathetic and compassion people also the most creative? Highly compassionate people care more about connections with people and therefore are more likely open to getting ideas from many different people that can combine into a creative thought. Their compassionate desire to help others also leads them to push themselves to go beyond the norm to really help the person and solve their problem. They creatively do more because they care more.

Sensory Intelligence. Finally, sensory intelligence is the third magic ingredient you will want in every member of you care team. Sensory intelligence is the ability to really tune into observing the environment. People with good sensory intelligence can see the subtleties of what is happening around them that others cannot. They see patterns to what is going on and when something is off. In this way by keenly observing their environment they are great at anticipating what will happen before it does.

You can see why this skill is so important for caregivers and physician care team members. You will want your caregivers to notice when something is not right with your loved one. They will notice if your loved one is acting different than usual. They may notice when your loved one is not feeling well or when they are sad or angry. This is very important.

They also may anticipate if your loved one is at any safety risk by noticing something off about your loved one's physical environment and how what your loved one is doing might cause a safety risk. A person with high sensory intelligence will anticipate these things very well. Perhaps the greatest professional hockey player of all time, Wayne Gretzky ("the Great Gretzky") used to say that he was successful because he would skate to where he thought the puck was going to be. His sensory intelligence, combined with his experience, helped him see patterns that no one else could see and could therefore anticipate where the puck was going to be. This is key for physicians too. Granneman and Solo found that physicians who had this high sensory intelligence were better because physicians because they could see patterns of symptoms and anticipate what was going to happen with a patient better than physicians without high sensory intelligence.

You can see how these three magic underlying traits are linked together. If you are highly empathetic and care more about others, you will be more creative because your connections with others will bring you more ideas; and you will want to use this information to go creatively deeper to solve others' problems. You will also have more sensory intelligence because your higher sensitivity will lead you to notice things others can't notice and your creativity will help you combine what you see in new ways that help you anticipate and solve problems in novel ways before they happen. These three traits can be so powerfully important for your loved one; you will want your entire care team to be stacked with people with these magical skills. You must find these remarkable people, but you also must lead them effectively to unleash these superpowers for your loved one.

Leading Team Members Who Have Compassion, Creativity, and Sensory Intelligence

The good news is that, if you find experienced and competent care team members with compassion, creativity, and sensory intelligence, they are relatively simple to lead. Granneman and Solo found these highly responsive and sensitive people to be driven by the importance of the purpose and meaning in what they are doing. When I shared that our mission was to help Mom live longer, healthier, and happier, I could see in our caregivers' eyes that they were inspired and motivated to do their very best. The importance of truly helping Mom self-activated their empathy, creativity, and sensory intelligence. They were driven by the power and meaning of this mission. They also saw my sister's and my commitment to both Mom and to them as Mom's caregivers. I would point them in the right direction with our clear mission and with clear expectations (outlined in Ch. 14) and then support, recognize, and appreciate them. They did amazing work and stayed with us for years and years.

In Chapter 12, I will share how I interviewed caregivers to look for these three superpowers and how I led these remarkable people in Chapter 13. I will also help you assess your medical team for these three superpowers in Chapter 20.

Finding Superpowered Caregivers

When I started thinking about getting caregiving help at home, I dusted off Mom's long term care insurance policy and saw that I needed to use an agency that had licensed caregivers to be reimbursed for care expenses. In retrospect, I am glad I used agencies; they were remarkable partners in helping me find the best care team for Mom.

I was a little concerned because I was not sure how Mom would accept a stranger coming into the house to take care of her. So, I wanted to start small and ease Mom into the idea of another person, other than my sister or I, caring for her. I called a few local home care agencies to learn about their policies and their experience with Alzheimer's patients. I quickly learned some agencies were comfortable with trial short care shifts and some not. Since I had no experience with hiring caregivers, I wanted to start the caregiver with a short shift to see how it would work out.

I wanted the agency to narrow down their caregiver possibilities to the 2-3 top candidates, whom I then wanted to interview before anyone came to our home. I told the agency that talking to these top 2-3 candidates was a "meeting with them," but it was really a selection interview. I would meet them at a local coffee shop for the interview. Even though I had interviewed many people in my human resources role, I had never interviewed a caregiver. To increase your chances of finding superpowered caregivers for your loved one, I strongly suggest you meet and hold a short selection interview. Most agencies are probably not used to the client asking to interview caregivers; the agency usually just sends a caregiver to your home or facility for the shift. I found it easier to tell the agency that I wanted to chat with a possible candidate first.

A good agency will ask you what you are looking for. A less than good agency will just send someone. To help the agency choose candidates that are a better fit for you and your loved one, give them a sense of the kind of person you are looking for and the hours and days you would like them to work. I knew I wanted caregivers with Alzheimer's or dementia experience who were warm, loving, and caring. When I gained more experience about what good and bad caregiving looked like, I refined what was important to me. I added things like being creative and compassionate, able to make interacting with Mom a fun experience, flexibility, experience with implementation of important safety protocols, and being really tuned into what was going on with Mom. All became very important for me. This list of caregiver expectations is in Chapter 14.

As a former HR executive, I knew even the best interviewing is not an exact science. I knew you really don't know someone until you see them on the job. After the interview, if I liked them, I wanted the person to work a short 3–4-hour shift to see how they worked with Mom and how Mom reacted to them before committing to longer shifts and more days.

We were taking care of Mom at home, but families who have their loved one in a facility often hire private caregivers to give their loved one 1:1 attention in a facility. This private care is often very important especially if the facility has a high patient to caregiver ratio. The method of selecting caregivers I describe here will work whether the caregivers are in the home or in a facility.

If a caregiver is just average, the Breakthrough Care System will not be implemented at a high enough level to extend your loved one's happiness or longevity. This is why interviewing and finding the finest is so vital. I did not know this in the beginning, but I benefitted greatly by having several agencies involved in helping me find these incredible caregivers. Working with several home healthcare agencies significantly increases the likelihood of finding the best caregivers.

Like workers in every field, a caregiver's capability ranges from poor to average to good to incredible. You can find better caregivers and more flexibility in shift coverage when you choose from more agencies because you will have a bigger pool of caregiver candidates to choose from.

Having several agencies to choose from will also be helpful when you need to find other resources your loved one will need. I found, over time, I needed someone to cut Mom's hair at our home. I also needed an at-home podiatrist, an at-home physical therapist, and eventually an at-home dentist. Home agencies helped me find all these people, and certain agencies had more experience with one kind of specialty versus another.

Caregiving agencies are also helpful because they are responsible, not you, for the human resources administration of your caregivers. The home care agencies do the background checking, provide health insurance, do the payroll, and help you with scheduling. Also, when you want to let go of a caregiver, all you do is tell the agency that the person is not a fit, and they will handle the rest. Home care agencies are a very important part of your care team.

Selection Interview Guide for Empowered Care Leaders

Where to Interview: I suggest you interview somewhere it will be quiet, and you won't be interrupted. I don't suggest you interview the caregiver for the first time at your home or in front of your loved one. With several people being considered, you may confuse and disorient your loved one with too many different people coming in the home. I interviewed at a local Starbucks during a time of the day when it was not busy.

Length of Time for the Selection Interview: Forty-five minutes is roughly the time needed to find out whether the candidate is a good fit for your loved one. If you are interviewing more than one person at the same location, I don't suggest you schedule them back-to-back. You will want to leave a little time between interviews in case you go a little longer with one candidate. In the minutes in between my interviews, I usually reviewed my notes and reflected on what I had learned about the caregiver candidate.

Structure of the Selection Interview

Step 1: Establish Rapport and Get Them Comfortable (warm-up) – (5-8 minutes)

Having a little small talk makes your candidate more comfortable, which usually results in a better interview. A comfortable candidate is likely to give you better information about themselves. You can ask them about their week or day or if they had any trouble getting to the location. You can also ask them an open-ended question like "tell me a little bit about yourself" or "tell me what you like about caregiving." These kinds of questions get them talking and will likely give you an initial sense about what kind of a person they are and what is important to them.

I would then tell them a little bit about myself, why I took an early retirement to take care of Mom, and other basic small talk. Finally, in this warm-up I would tell them a small amount about Mom, like when she was diagnosed with Alzheimer's and about her career as a kindergarten teacher. I purposely do not tell the candidate too much about Mom at this early juncture. If I tell them all about Mom, they may not feel they need to ask about her. I learn a lot about the candidate by what questions the candidate asks about Mom. If they ask nothing about Mom, it often means the candidate is not very caring, not motivated, or lacks intellectual curiosity about her habits, behavior, or routine. If the candidate asks what the kinds of games or activities Mom likes most, it indicates that the candidate knows how important stimulation is for Mom and her disease. It also indicates that she is sensitive to what Mom wants to do.

Step 2: Core of the Interview: What they Do in Care Situations (25 minutes)

Interviewing is not nearly as effective as seeing the candidate on the job. However, you can get an idea of what the candidate is like on the job by asking them "in action" questions. For example, "tell me about a time a dementia patient was particularly challenging; what specifically did you do?". This question gives me an idea of what a caregiver finds particularly challenging and what actions and thought processes they use in a particular situation. As an example, a candidate might say "my patient ignored what I asked them to do." If the caregiver seemed frustrated about that and could not find a solution, I would consider that candidate not adequate as Mom's caregiver. If they said, "I convinced her she needed a shower," then I would ask "how did you do that?" If it sounded like they bullied the patient and did not come up with a creative fun diversionary way, such as a game, or other creative method to get the patient into the shower, they are not a good fit with my high expectations for a creative, caring, and fun caregiver. If the candidate expresses any frustration with the patient, they are not nearly as empathetic, compassionate, or skilled as they need to be.

Mastering the art of compassionately and creatively redirecting the dementia patient and having fun are important tools for good dementia caregiving. "Redirecting" is acknowledging the patient's feelings or wants, agreeing with their perspective (not criticizing or telling them they are wrong), and creatively changing the subject or the focus from what is troubling the patient to something they like, returning later to what the caregiver wants the patient to do. In the case of a patient resisting a shower, the kind of creative care answer to "what did you do or say when they resisted the shower?" is: "I know you don't want a shower now, I completely understand that, no problem, let's play with this stuffed animal for a while," or "let's look at this magazine instead". Then, when the patient is less resistant, a superpowered caregiver would come back to the shower idea and reassure the patient that everything is OK and that they will have fun in the shower. This is a great way to get a noncompliant loved one with dementia to work with the caregiver and not against him or her. This is the same way you might guide a child. Other than keeping your loved one "safe", it is not often necessary for the patient to do what the caregiver wants at that specific moment (there is always time for the activity later when the patient is calmer and more compliant). If the candidate in the interview talks about making things fun and comfortable for your loved one, you may have a remarkable caregiver candidate. Creating a fun activity for your loved one like singing a silly song or telling a story with a stuffed animal or doll to comfort a patient are how I wanted my potential caregiver to approach Mom with if she was resistant.

Another subtle caregiving skill to watch for in the interview that shows savvy is the "yes… and." Good caregivers don't disagree, criticize, tell their patients they are wrong, tell them they already told them that, or test dementia patients. They know how to use the "yes….and" technique. The dementia patient may complain or stubbornly disagree with the caregiver. The skilled caregiver will agree with the dementia patient ("Yes!"), compassionately understand them, and then say what they want to say. Good caregivers rarely use the words "no," "you are wrong" or "but"; "yes… and" shows this savvy understanding on the part of your caregiver candidate.

Don't be afraid to ask probing questions to go deeper and find out how your potential caregiver handled any challenging situation. If the candidate says that they never had trouble with an Alzheimer's patient, they either are not telling the truth or never actively engaged their patient in doing the kinds of things you will want them to do. The more real-life samples of the candidate's behavior you ask for the better picture you will have of the caregiver's interaction with your loved one. With good interviewing techniques, I was able to filter out a lot of poor and average caregivers who didn't have the experience or superpower care skills I was looking for.

Step 3: Answer the Interviewee's Questions (10 minutes)

Answer any questions the caregiver candidate may have. Once again, I learned the most about the candidate by the questions they asked. For example, one potential caregiver asked, "is your mom incontinent?" or "does your mom yell a lot?" The potential caregiver's question may signal that they don't like these kinds of behaviors or worse they won't handle them well or at all. A question like that is a yellow flag for you to probe a little deeper. However, if your potential caregiver asks: "what does your mom like to do?" then that is a good sign from your candidate. It may mean that the candidate places a high priority on meeting your loved one's needs and will be creative in stimulating your loved one. I like candidates to ask me good thoughtful questions. If they don't ask any questions at all, I probably won' hire that candidate because it could be that they are not motivated or creative enough for what I want them to do with Mom.

Step 4: Closing the Interview & Next Steps (3 – 5 minutes)

Thank them for the time they spent with you and tell them what the next steps will be. Give them a rough timeline about when you will be making your decision and tell them that you will get back to the agency. If you like them and are seriously considering them, then tell them what you liked about them. They may have a choice about where to work (especially if they are as good as you need them to be) and that can get them more motivated to work for you. If you did not like the candidate, the agency will handle the rejection for you.

Post-Interview Reflection

Reflect on notes you took during the interview and your impressions about how the candidate would fit or not fit with your loved one. The agency should have done reference checks; you can find out from the agency what prior clients specifically said about the caregiver candidate. If the agency did not do reference checks or doesn't know much about the candidate, that may be a signal to look for another agency.

If you liked the caregiver and felt positive about hiring this candidate, compare them with other strong candidates you have seen. If after reflecting on the interview you still find missing pieces, ask the agency if they have any information that might shed light on anything about the candidate you are still wondering about. The agency is your partner to help you identify the very best candidates.

I am confident anyone can do this kind of selection interview. It is perfectly fine to look down and refer to your notes or a list of questions and probes to remind what you are looking do in the interview. Like anything, the first time or two you do this kind of interview you might feel a little uncomfortable, but you will get better each time you do one.

Selection interviewing is an important life skill. Remember, if I can do it, so can you!

Don't settle for just anyone. Your loved one deserves someone who deeply cares about safety first, is empathetic and creative, will have fun with them, and will not cause angst or put pressure on your loved one in any way. If you are not totally sure about hiring the candidate but you do like certain things about the caregiver, try them out on a short shift and see how they do and how your loved one responds to them. If you think the group of candidates a particular agency provided are overall not meeting your expectations, get a different agency to provide candidates.

Evaluating a New Caregiver

You are building a high-powered A+ Care Team. I wanted our caregivers to feel that it is a privilege to be on Team Mom. As care leader, I was accountable to be sure everyone did a top-notch job. Great sourcing from a strong agency and good selection interviewing was an essential foundation.

The concept of *"Situational Leadership"* applies here. Simply put, when someone is inexperienced, either working in a new situation or inexperienced overall, they will need more structure, guidance, and supervision. As their experience grows and they become more capable in the new situation, the leader can safely back off and provide less guidance and supervision. Since my new caregivers were experienced but in a new situation taking care of Mom, I followed situational leadership principles: I observed and guided them more in the beginning. Then, when I saw the caregiver was doing well, I would step back but support them as they did their magic with Mom.

In the beginning phase when I was supervising more directly, I watched out especially for Mom's safety and how the caregiver was establishing rapport and engaging Mom. When the new caregiver transferred Mom from the bed, chair, or toilet to standing and to the walker, I always watched for how safely they did this. Transferring is the time when there is the biggest risk of falling. An experienced caregiver knows how important it is to transfer a patient safely. Experienced and compassionate caregivers know how to do this. Our caregivers knew the best techniques for lifting Mom to keep her safe. A good caregiver would ask Mom to put her hands around their neck; they would then put their hands around Mom's mid-section and then use their legs to lift Mom up safely. Mom was only 5' 2", but for any body type, this is the correct way to lift your loved one. Thankfully, Mom was usually very cooperative when our caregivers would transfer her correctly from sitting to standing. I noticed that Mom would resist when a caregiver was not doing it correctly. Since Mom could not talk, I'm guessing Mom must not have felt safe or maybe did not like the caregiver and that may be why she resisted. One potential caregiver asked if I had a "transfer belt" for Mom. A transfer belt is a wide belt that can be fastened around the patient's hips and pulled by the caregiver to help lift the patient. I had one to use at home, but I found it a little slow to put on and extremely cumbersome to use. If a caregiver knew what they were doing, it didn't look like it was necessary to use a transfer belt. The combination of the caregiver holding Mom around the waist and Mom's hands around the caregiver's neck was a more comforting, loving, positive, and safer experience for Mom. I understand transfer belts themselves can cause injury. To me, it was a little like a flight attendant asking you to put on a parachute when you are boarding your flight… it may be safe but overkill for the situation. This brand-new caregiver did not want to lift Mom any other way. Because she was so inflexible and not as creatively capable as other potential caregivers, I did not ask her back.

When Mom started walking down the hall of our home, I accompanied new caregivers to see how Mom and they handled the walker. Because Mom was wobbly and a little off balance when walking sometimes, she was at risk of falling. The caregiver needed to concentrate and behave a little more seriously when walking with Mom, so Mom was less distracted while walking. I noticed that the best caregivers knew how important walking without distractions was and would always gently place Mom's hands on the walker before their walk started. Also, our caregiver would walk along with Mom while holding the walker from the front end. Some would gently hold both of Mom's hands onto the handles of the walker so Mom would always be holding the walker. Occasionally, Mom did take her hands off the walker. If the caregiver was not holding onto her hands, Mom might have fallen backwards. The other approach that seemed even safer was where one of the caregivers' hands would hold one of Mom's hands on the walker and then the other hand was around Mom's back as they walked together. Both methods seemed effective, but the latter approach seemed even safer to me. If a new caregiver did not do either and let Mom just walk on her own with the walker, I would intervene and show them this technique that I learned from the outstanding caregivers. If after explaining how I wanted them to use the walker, if I saw later in the shift the caregiver reverting to not holding Mom while walking, she was not the right caregiver for us.

I also always observed closely when getting to know a new caregiver how well the new caregiver was connecting with Mom, having fun, and building rapport with her. I watched how and if Mom responded to the caregiver. On the caregiver's first day, I would introduce them to Mom and tell Mom that a new caregiver was going to help today. I would remind the caregiver that Mom had lost her speech. Occasionally, a new caregiver was completely clueless on how to connect with Mom because she was not able to speak. Mom always had the ability to give you a big smile and communicate with her eyes and expressions. If Mom was having fun and liked you, you could see it in her face. A good caregiver would figure out Mom's way of communicating. The good caregivers would give Mom a big smile and Mom would smile big back. Mom was so adorable because she would gesture to the caregivers she liked with her finger, indicating that she wanted them to come close to her; then Mom would give the caregiver a big hug and plant a big noisy kiss on their cheek.

The creative empathetic caregivers might notice something Mom was wearing and tell her how pretty it was. Since Mom was a girl, I've been told by her childhood friends, she always liked dressing nicely and was proud of her sense of style. Her love of dressing up and style did not change during her Alzheimer's journey. The good caregivers learned that Mom loved to look in her mirror to see what she had on. Caregivers noticed that when they were helping Mom dress, she always wanted to wear something that matched and was tasteful and in style. They also figured out that when they made funny faces in the bathroom mirror, Mom would make funny faces back at them and laugh just like a child. Mom also liked to watch the caregiver put lipstick and powder on her in the mirror. The top-notch caregivers knew how to have fun with Mom from the beginning and played creative games with her and her favorite dolls and stuffed animals.

If the caregiver was calm and having fun, then Mom was calm and having fun. If the caregiver was nervous and telling Mom what to do, she would then not cooperate or would look sad. I noticed that before Mom would follow a caregiver's direction, she would have to feel a connection with her and like her. If she liked the caregiver, she would usually smile and do whatever the caregiver asked of her.

There were some unacceptable new caregivers who would just sit on the chair and watch TV or check their i-Phones; they were detached and even seemed bored and disinterested. To me, these "drones" did not want to do the work to connect, stimulate, and have fun with Mom. I don't know if these incompetent caregivers just thought that their job was only to respond to Mom if she needed or wanted something. I expected a lot more of Mom's caregivers; they needed to be proactive in creating fun and stimulating activities to keep Mom active and engaged. When the caregiver would rather find anything to do rather than connecting and creatively stimulating Mom, I knew this was not the right caregiver for her. These drones might straighten out Mom's room or her clothes, check their cell phone every five minutes, or just sit quietly next to Mom without saying a word. I was crystal clear and let a new caregiver know that the two most important parts of their job were safety and creatively having fun and connecting with Mom. If I felt Mom was not 100% safe and noticed any risk of a fall or an injury, I would not invite them to do another shift. However, if I saw a spark of connection and some creativity to stimulate Mom and their safety skills were solid, I would ask them back and observe them on the creative connecting fun part on their second shift.

It was wonderful to see how a superpowered caregiver would have wonderful communication with Mom even though she did not speak any words. Mom understood almost everything said to her but just could not respond with words. The good caregivers figured out how to communicate with Mom. Our remarkable caregivers would tease and joke with Mom and use their cellphones to play music from the 50's which she enjoyed. Since Mom grew up in New York in the 50's with many fellow Italian friends, she would smile and was delighted to hear her songs from Frank Sinatra, Tony Bennet, Doris Day, and many favorite nostalgic 50's songs. Her caregivers would draw pictures while Mom was drawing pictures; Mom was always polite because she never let on that she probably thought the caregiver's drawing was not as good as hers. Mom was always smiling and happy with her incredible caregivers. They would read stories to Mom, especially "children's" stories because Mom was a kindergarten teacher for so many years. I am so glad we found such wonderful caregivers because they worked with Mom so well and made the time with her so special. They loved their jobs and never just sat on a chair "to put in their time." I wanted Mom to live longer and happier; regular, proactive, and creative fun and activity is mission-critical for this purpose.

If you live in an urban or suburban area, there are dozens of agencies and hundreds of caregivers to choose from for your loved one. Please, don't settle for an average caregiver. The very best caregivers will bring this special spark to your loved one. When you see the joy your loved one will have with these very special caregivers, you will feel joy, too. I believe you will find doing your selection interviews and observing a new caregiver's skills on a trial shift will be well worth your investment of time and energy. Finding superpowered caregivers pays big dividends to your loved and will provide you the gift of time and peace of mind. You will know these superstars are taking great care of your loved one.

When to Immediately Fire a New Caregiver

Sometimes, you will need to observe a new caregiver for a couple of shifts to see if they have the skills and attitude to become an A+ caregiver for your loved one. In Chapter 13, I will share how to coach caregivers. The purpose of coaching is to turn very good caregivers into incredibly great caregivers.

Tragically, you might see some behaviors from a new caregiver that are so unsafe, so dangerous, or so far from what you are trying to achieve that you must fire them immediately. These situations are:

Sleeping On the Job

To help me be an effective care leader and manage Mom's entire Care System, I needed sleep. To do this, the first shift I wanted help with was the overnight shift. Mom needed a lot of care during the night. For a person with Alzheimer's, nighttime can sometimes be the most difficult and challenging times for both patient and caregiver. Many Alzheimer's and dementia patients have what is called Sundowners Syndrome. This makes it difficult for Alzheimer's patients to sleep at night, and they become restless and agitated at times. Mom was so happy at home that I don't think I would call her agitated. She did, however, tend to be active and a little restless at night. Our great caregivers were smart and had observed her well enough to know when she was ready to sleep at night and when having fun and playing was much more comforting for her. Therefore, nighttime is often the time for a caregiver to be extra diligent, careful, and extra creative.

I was trying out a new caregiver for an overnight shift. Her first overnight shift went all right. On her second overnight shift, I was sleeping in the room next door, and I heard a loud bang coming from Mom's room. I ran into Mom's room and saw Mom flat on the floor. I was petrified that she had been injured and asked the new caregiver what happened! She told me that Mom had gotten up so fast, scooting down and slipping out the bottom of the bed (no rail at the foot of the bed) that she had had no time to get over to the bed to stop Mom's fall. This excuse was stupid. If she was really watching Mom, she would have seen her trying to get up and out of the bed and would have been right there to help her up. This was the first and only time in Mom's long journey that she had ever fallen. My sister and I were not only angry but very worried about Mom. As I carefully lifted Mom up from the soft rug, I checked to see if she was in pain or if she had broken her leg or arm, or her head or face. It did not appear she had broken anything or was in pain. My sister and I knew that God was looking out for us that night. I had put rubber guards on all the furniture edges in her room and saw that one of these rubber guards prevented her from getting seriously hurt. She did have a few bruises and a black eye but nothing that needed immediate emergency attention. I obviously immediately sent this caregiver home.

The next day we took Mom to the doctor to get checked out, and other than a few bruises and her black eye, she was in good shape. I looked at the video from my mom's nighttime room camera. As a side note, cameras are legal to use if you don't tape sound and if you don't place them in any of the caregiver's private areas (for example their bathroom or where they sleep). I used the room camera only to evaluate new caregivers for overnight shifts because I was sleeping and could not observe. The cameras are very easy to use and inexpensive. I am so glad I had the camera going because the tape clearly showed that this caregiver had fallen asleep on the floor instead of being awake and helping Mom. It showed Mom had scooted herself down to the bottom part of the bed and tried to get up! It took a good amount of time for Mom to scoot down and position herself at the bottom part of the bed. The caregiver had no idea what was happening because she was sound asleep. I told the agency what happened, and I hope she will never work for anyone again.

Lengthy Phone Use

Cell phones, now in widespread use, can easily be a big distraction for a caregiver. Great caregivers never get bored on the job, and so they rarely look at their phones. The best caregivers take pride in their profession and understand the importance of keeping your loved one safe, stimulated, and given a lot of attention and love. Most great caregivers see their role as the special privilege it is. The less-than-stellar caregivers revert to their phone for their own stimulation and entertainment. You can identify a poor caregiver when you see them making lengthy calls or spending time texting or playing games on their phone. I totally understand if they must use their phone for a personal emergency or to quickly check to see if their child or family member is okay. However, a caregiver's phone use is a major distraction that puts the mission of providing safety, love, and creative stimulation in jeopardy.

When I reviewed the tape for another new overnight caregiver who spent hours talking to someone on the phone, it looked like Mom was awake, sitting up, and wanted to interact and play with the caregiver; however, this caregiver completely ignored Mom and was more interested in talking on the phone. A caregiver who is more interested in long talks on the phone rather than interacting and stimulating Mom has no place on Team Mom and is not a caregiver for your loved one, either. These thoughtless, dangerous caregivers need to be let go quickly.

Drugs or Alcohol Use

Drugs or alcohol use among your caregivers should not be tolerated and the use of these substances should not be used before or during a shift. My mom had a new caregiver who seemed kind and attentive on her first shift, but by her second shift, she looked to me like she was struggling to talk and complete any task. To me, on the second shift she looked like a completely different person. I was puzzled and didn't know what was wrong. I was very worried Mom would be in danger of a fall so I told her to tidy up Mom's clean laundry in the living room and that I would take care of Mom for a while.

After a short time, I asked Marina to be with Mom, and I went into the living room to see what she was doing. She had been folding laundry in the living room for 45 minutes and had only folded three small bath towels. She wasn't asleep but was incoherent and somewhat confused. I asked her what was wrong and if she was ill. To her credit, she was honest; she told me that just before her shift she had been "huffing." I do not know much about drugs, so I googled this term and was shocked to find out it means to "inhale the vapors of some drug in order to become intoxicated." After that, I knew if she stayed, Mom would be in danger and sent her home immediately.

I know the home care agencies screen their caregivers for drugs and alcohol, but like selection interviewing, drug screening is not always done regularly. From that day forward, I kept an eye out for any sign of intoxication with new caregivers. I did feel sorry for this young lady, and I prayed that she could end her addiction. However, our loved one's safety and happiness are too important to ignore any sign that a caregiver is unable to function at the very top of their game while working with our loved ones. Caregiving done at a breakthrough level is a very demanding job and takes tremendous concentration, empathy, and creativity. You and your loved one deserve the best care, and you should not tolerate any of these compromising behaviors from anyone.

After a few shifts, and discovering they had the baseline motivation, skills, and high standards, and were loving, compassionate, and creative people with no "knockout" factors (e.g., drugs, excessive phone use, sleeping on the job, or just sitting and doing nothing), I was ready to introduce the selected caregivers to my "Caregiver Expectations List." My Expectations List is the list of very specific behaviors that I want and expect Mom's caregivers to follow. These specific expectations are the detailed methods that the caregiver must execute to activate the Breakthrough Care System for Mom on every shift. In Chapter 14, I will detail for you this list of expectations that I created as I learned over time.

Chapter Summary

1. Use caregiving agencies, especially if you are a new care leader. Agencies can help you find great caregivers. The caregiver really works for you, but technically they work for the agency, so the agency handles benefits, payroll, and termination. Use several agencies to expand your pool of caregiving talent and other

resources you may need. Home care agencies are your wonderful partners and key members of your care team.

2.   Interview the top couple of candidates from the best agencies. Think about what you'll need from the candidate before the interview. Think about the days and hours you need as well as skills and personal traits you want. This chapter includes suggestions on effective skills and traits to look for. Even more specifics of what to look for in the selection interview are in my List of Caregiver Expectations detailed in Chapter 14.

3.   Use the *"Care Leader's Caregiver Selection Interview Guide"* in this chapter to interview caregiver candidates. This interview guide builds off a proven interview method to give you confidence and help you rule out caregivers who don't have the desired superpowers. If it is awkward in the beginning, keep using it; it will get easier for you.

4.   Don't settle for average caregivers. Keep your standards high to find the best candidates. You will need incredible caregivers to implement the high standards required for the Breakthrough Care System. Hold the home care agencies to high standards to find truly remarkable candidates for you. You and your loved one will benefit so much by keeping your standards very high.

5.   If after interviewing, you like a candidate, then set up a tryout for a short shift. If you identify serious safety issues or behavioral problems, immediately call the agency and tell them you don't want the person anymore. If you observe them doing a wonderful job of keeping your loved one safe and have a great connection and creatively stimulating your loved one, you may be fortunate enough to have found a game-changing caregiver.

CHAPTER 13

Leading Remarkable Caregivers Once You Have Found Them

I was a novice when I began the journey with Mom. However, with hunger to learn, I observed Mom's care and learned a lot about her unique needs as an Alzheimer's patient. As I learned from the good caregivers and seeing Mom's responses to our caregivers, I began to write down my insights about what seemed to work best with Mom. I began to turn these insights into a list of specific expectations for myself and for each of our caregivers. This list, which I will share in the next chapter, became my baseline to coach caregivers and to recognize my caregivers when they met these expectations exceptionally well. My very best caregivers did most of the items on the *Caregivers Expectations List* very naturally. A caregiver may be outstanding overall but on occasion may have a lapse in an area or two. In these cases, the following coaching approach worked well to keep everyone caring for Mom at the highest level.

The Care Leader's Coaching for Improvement Guide

I learned this basic method of coaching early in my human resources career. The basic structure of this coaching guide works for all coaching situations. I found it worked well for coaching Mom's care team. Once you find your remarkable caregivers, this coaching method can help turn your very good caregivers into truly remarkable caregivers. First, I will share the coaching method, and then I will provide an actual example of a coaching conversation I had with one of Mom's caregivers.

Coaching for Improvement: Steps

1. Identify the Gap in Performance: "The Problem" (the difference between expectation and what happened)

The first step is to make sure the caregiver knows where they have fallen short of the expectation you have of them. The performance gap is the difference between what you expect of them and their actual performance in a situation. If you can get the caregiver to tell you what they did incorrectly, they will remember it better and be more likely to have a feeling of ownership for the solution. You do this by asking them a question designed to get them to tell you what they did incorrectly. It is also important not to wait too long to have the coaching conversation. If you wait too long, you and the caregiver may forget important details of what happened. You can ask a "what" question to identify what did not go so well. The question might be something like "What happened?" or "What might have gone better?".

2. Clarify the Root Cause of This Gap in Performance

Understanding why this performance gap or performance problem happened is critical to finding the solution. There may be many reasons performance does not happen the way you expect it. It could be a training issue, or maybe the caregiver did not know it was a priority. Questions that get to the root cause are usually "why?" questions. For example, "Why do you think that happened?". If you want to go a little deeper after you get the answer to "Why do you think this happened," you could ask "Why do you think this is?" These questions will get to the cause of the problem. Then, follow with a shift to finding a solution, using questions like "What things could you have done differently to avoid this?". Focusing on the "why" and "alternative solutions" gets to solving the problem rather than assigning blame. A problem-solving line of questions reduces the likelihood of a defensive unproductive reaction from the caregiver.

3. Zero In on the Solution to Close the Performance Gap

Once again, it is better if the caregiver identifies the solution to the performance problem. This builds their sense of ownership (makes them feel more responsible), fueling resolve to avoid the performance gap going forward. After your alternative solutions question can ask, "Of these possible solutions, to avoid this problem in the future, which solution would work best in your mind"? Then, to help build the caregiver's commitment to that solution, you can ask, "Why do you think that would be the best solution?"

4. Identify What Will Make the Solution Sustainable

Ask what the caregiver needs to ensure the solution will work and be sustainable. Ask a question like, "what do you think will really make this solution work?" They may be able to identify the solution but something else may be inhibiting them from it working longer term. For example, if the caregiver thinks they have too many duties that need to be done at the same time, they may need help in prioritizing or help eliminating a task to make the solution work. To avoid these unexpected barriers to the solution working, ask a question like, "Is there anything that might get in the way of this solution working in the short and long term?"

A Real Caregiver Coaching Example

If the caregiver has too many performance issues coaching may not help. You may simply want to find a different caregiver. But if the caregiver is very good overall but has a specific area that could get a little better, then you will be able to coach them to improve in that area; this kind of coaching conversation doesn't take much time and with a caregiver who wants to be great it usually solves the problem.

We had a caregiver that was overall excellent and very loving, creative, and compassionate. She had great fun with Mom, and Mom responded to her beautifully. Our caregiver was very solid on safety behaviors but there was a situation when there was a momentary lapse when Mom was walking with her walker into the garage to get into the car to go out on one of our daily adventures. There was a safety lapse that was not acceptable and would benefit from coaching. Mom's safety is everything because all it takes is a momentary lapse to have a huge problem. With safety I believe there is zero room for error. In this coaching example, Mom was transitioning from her walker to getting into the car and she almost fell. My sister Marina was there thankfully and immediately got up against our mom and stopped her from falling. With this almost falling example, after we got home, I asked this caregiver to take a couple of minutes with me; Marina took care of Mom while I took a moment to coach the caregiver.

The coaching for improvement conversation went like this:

Mark: "When Mom was getting into the car a little while ago Marina mentioned that you had a problem with Mom when she was getting into the car. What happened?

Caregiver: "Lena [Mom] almost fell transitioning into the car".

Mark: "You know we don't want any falling, right?"

Caregiver: "Yes, of course."

Mark: "Why do you think this happened?"

Caregiver: "I think the walker was too far away from the open car door when your mom started to get into the car. I should have made sure she was closer to the car."

Mark: "Were there any other reasons?"

Caregiver: "I turned my back to your mom to straighten out the car seat pad before she got in."

Mark: "How might you have done this differently?"

Caregiver: "First, I could have had your mom walk closer to the car door with the walker before we started getting in."

Mark: "Good. Anything else?"

Caregiver: "I also could have asked Marina to hold your mom while I straightened the car seat. Or, I could have asked Marina to straighten out the car seat while I held onto your mom."

Mark: "Yes! good! This sound like it would have worked much better. I'm sure you know it only takes a moment for my mom to have a serious fall."

Caregiver: "Yep!"

Mark: "Is there anything I can do to help you keep my mom safe in this kind of situation?"

Caregiver: "No, I don't think so. It is great that you and Marina come on our outings; it helps me a lot. I should remember to ask you guys for your help when I need it. "

Mark: "Yes, exactly, we are a team. That's one reason we come with you on our outings because we help each other to make it a fun and safe for Mom. You do a great job with Mom. Mom loves being with you. You have so much fun and have such a great connection with her; we come along to help and support. It is important that you always ask for help or anything else you need to help Mom. We want her to be 100% safe and for everyone to have fun. I hope you know you are very important to Mom and to Marina and to me. Thank you for being so open to talking about this; I really appreciate it."

This simple coaching conversation only took about five minutes. With the right method and a caring attitude, the conversation went well and maintained this important caregiver's self-esteem. It also seemed to get to the root cause of the problem. The caregiver needed to think ahead a bit more and ask for help when she needed it. Also, she needed a reminder that safety and not falling needed to be put higher in her priorities. My sister and I really love and cared about this caregiver and felt she was a very important part of Mom's Care Team. I really wanted her to be successful for both Mom and for us. I used the conversation as an opportunity to reinforce how important fall prevention is for Mom, to think ahead and anticipate problems, and to reinforce the fact that Marina or I are always nearby and want to help. Also, I wanted her to know that asking us for help is a strength not a weakness. I think our caregiver was reminded that all of us working together can be a powerful team.

Like the *Caregiver Selection Interviewing Guide* in Chapter 12, this *Caregiver Coaching for Improvement Guide* may be a little awkward the first time you try it, but it gets easier. I encourage you to ask the coaching questions in your own voice, the same way you would say anything. The main thing is getting to the root cause of the problem and to come up with a solution that is sustainable over time and that can be committed to. For many people, including me, confronting people is hard. I am conflict-averse. By initiating this caregiver coaching, you are not being a jerk with your caregivers, you are being professional and protecting your loved one. Excellent caregivers want to be successful. Reframe coaching as helping the caregiver go from being good to great. Your caregivers are highly motivated and want to be incredible to achieve the breakthrough longevity and happiness mission. You will also have peace of mind knowing your loved one is being taken care of by remarkably great caregivers. Remember, keeping your expectations high will help your loved one live longer, healthier, and happier. Like the selection interview method, this coaching method is a life skill that can benefit you in many areas.

Chapter Summary

1. Once you have brought on strong caregivers on your team by using the selection interviewing methods in Chapter 12, following a professional coaching method like the one in this chapter can take your strong caregiver and make them superstars.

2. First, you must have a clear idea of what you expect of your team members. In Chapter14 there is a list of important caregiver expectations to work from. These are the expectations that are tied to helping your loved one live healthier, happier, and longer.

3. Second, you need to observe your caregivers in action to see if they are meeting your expectations.

4. Then if they are not meeting each expectation, follow this chapter's detailed coaching method. This method is a tried-and-true method to help the caregiver and you get to the root cause of any gap in performance. The method will also maintain the self-esteem of the caregiver and make you look good too.

5. You will be an outstanding care leader when you clarify your high expectations, coach each caregiver to achieve each expectation at the highest level. You, the caregiver and your loved one will benefit from your work in this area. It may take a little practice and feel a little awkward at first, but the effort will pay off for you and your loved one.

CHAPTER 14

The Empowered Care Leader's Expectations List

My list of caregiver expectations evolved over time by observing and learning what was important for my mom and what our exceptional caregivers did. This list applied for Mom from the time we had caregivers throughout her Alzheimer's journey.

Your list will likely be very similar to mine, but it should be tailored to your loved one's specific needs. Because dementia is a little different for everyone, if you observe your loved one carefully you can learn the unique patterns of their needs. Your loved one has their own special emotional, personal, physical, and medical symptoms and needs. Building those special needs into your own unique list of expectations will help your loved one and you tremendously. Your list may also evolve a little based on the phase of dementia your loved one is in and the unique aspects their journey.

As I used this Expectations List to communicate my expectations of caregivers, coach them for improvement, and appreciate and recognize remarkable caregiving, Mom thrived as the power of Breakthrough Care at the highest level was activated through clear and realized expectations. Most of these caregiver expectations are self-explanatory; however, in some cases, after each one I've included a few notes that provide a little more context.

Caregiver Expectations: The Top 5 Priorities

1. Never let Mom fall or even have the remote risk of falling

How:

a. Keep *two hands* on Mom, holding her whenever she is on her feet standing or walking…. no matter what … no excuses. Always use the walker. Keep two hands on her even if she is using the walker. If you hold Mom in a kind and loving way, she won't resist your hands on her. Please, don't ever assume it is okay not to have hands on Mom when she is standing or walking.

b. If Mom is sitting, have your eyes on her 100% of the time, no matter what; don't be tempted by distractions. If you need to look away or get something, plan ahead; ask Marina or me to watch Mom. Do not step out of Mom's direct view at any time. Please, don't ever assume it is okay that she is not watched.

c. If Mom falls asleep in a chair, sit right next to her. Do not leave space between Mom and you. It is very easy for her to fall over and get hurt while she is asleep and sitting up in a chair.

Keynote: The why and how of not falling is fundamental. It is mostly about being hands on and really concentrating to avoid a fall for your loved one. Also, be sure the pathway does not have floppy throw rugs or objects like toys, towels, or anything else that can cause a fall. We have a very docile cat at home who never got in Mom's way, but a feisty cat or an excited dog could easily cause your loved one to fall. A pet can be a great comfort for your loved one, but really watch because they can also be a fall risk.

2. Make sure Mom does not choke on food or anything else

How:

a. Watch Mom 100% of the time so she does not put anything in her mouth that is not supposed to be there, like toys, jewelry, bites of food that are too big or too hard to chew or swallow.

Think ahead, anticipate, and ask yourself, "Is there something in this area that Mom might put in her mouth that she shouldn't?"

b. Make sure Mom has *completely swallowed her food* or drink before giving her anything new to eat or drink. How do you do this? Watch her throat while she swallows. You can tell when she has swallowed her food or drink when you see her throat move up and down.

c. Make sure Mom *eats and drinks very slowly*. Make sure she has chewed sufficiently. Make sure everything is cut up finely in small pieces, crushed, or liquified.

Keynote: Difficulty swallowing is very common for Alzheimer's patients. The medical term is dysphagia; *and it is a very common cause of aspiration pneumonia, choking, and death in Alzheimer's patients. My mom would tend to put things in her mouth. Swallowing issues are more common as your loved one's dementia advances. This can lead to aspiration pneumonia and happens due to your loved one inhaling food particles or liquids into the lung. Aspiration pneumonia is one of the leading causes of death in dementia patients. With humor and positive distraction, our great caregivers were creative in knowing how to both slow Mom down and have her still enjoy eating.*

3. Make sure you take Mom to the bathroom frequently and really clean her well so she never gets a UTI (Urinary Tract Infection).

How:

a. Clean Mom right away. Never let her sit in things she shouldn't be sitting in. Since Mom cannot speak, keenly observe the nonverbal clues from her to know when she wants to go to the bathroom. She may point to the bathroom, groan, or sigh, or may be more agitated than usual. Promptly take Mom to the bathroom as soon as you see one of these or other nonverbal clues.

b. Be sure to clean Mom carefully, thoroughly, and correctly.

Keynote: Women are highly prone to UTIs. A UTI can be dangerous for dementia patients. Because a UTI can cause confusion, agitation, depression, and sleep disturbance, it is hard to know if these behavioral issues are coming from worsening dementia or from a UTI. Dementia patients usually cannot express to you what they are feeling or pain they are feeling from a UTI or other condition. This can result in a delay in giving your loved one the necessary care, and that can lead to a serious bladder or kidney infection.

If your loved one lives in a facility and is fully or partially incontinent, it is important that your loved one be cared for properly and that any infection be promptly treated. Unfortunately, many facilities are understaffed so you may want to hire a private caregiver to stay with your loved one and take them to the bathroom frequently. If your loved one is not brought to the bathroom frequently enough, cleaned well, and remains wet or dirty for a period, your loved one will get frequent UTI's and could easily end up with damaged kidneys or even sepsis.

Also, because UTIs cause agitation and confusion, if your loved one with dementia is living in a facility and becomes highly agitated (due to a UTI), some facilities may not know it is a UTI and suggest a tranquilizer or sleeping pill to calm down the patient. These medications usually dangerously speed up the dementia process.

4. Give the right food, pills, vitamins and food supplements correctly 100% of the time

How:

a. *Really pay attention to the details of what you are doing.*

Does every pill in the weekly pill box that I give you look like the correct pill? Did you give her every pill that you are supposed to by the end of each meal?

b. If something does not look right, for example, if something is missing, it is important that you ask me about it. Ensuring that Mom safely takes all her pills and supplements is very important.

c. We don't want Mom to choke on a pill so make sure her mouth is clear before giving her an additional pill or additional food. Make sure she is taking the pill with lots of water, or place the pill in some apple sauce to help swallowing. Certain pills are big, and I will crush them for you to put in apple sauce.

Keynote: Because prescriptions, vitamins, supplements, and overall nutrition were so very important to me, I wanted to do most of Mom's meal preparation and prepare the weekly pill box. Our caregivers were responsible each day to make sure meals and pills were properly and safely administered to Mom. Another reason I did all the meal and pill prep was because I wanted the caregiver to be 100% focused on Mom's safety and her enjoyably eating and taking her medications. I wanted no distractions from this.

5. Make your shift as creatively stimulating, loving and as fun an experience as possible:

How:

a. *Have fun with Mom.* Use your sense of humor, your special personality, and creative spirit to have fun. Even though you are an adult, don't be afraid to be childlike with Mom. She taught kindergarten for many years and feels very comfortable communicating this way.

b. Initiate, create, and participate in stimulating and fun activities with her. Examples include reading stories, drawing pictures, singing, or listening to music, doing puzzles, or imaginatively playing with her dolls and stuffed animals. You can read to her or tell her what's in the newspaper or magazines. Use your imagination and initiative; keep Mom stimulated and engaged as much as you can.

c. Make Mom laugh and smile as much as you can. She has a great smile and loves to laugh; laughing really lifts her mood. Make it a personal goal for you to make her smile and laugh a lot on every shift. Think actively and creatively about what Mom likes to do most.

d. Focus on her. Give 100% of your attention to her, not to other people in the room, your cell phone, the television, straightening things out, or any other "distraction."

e. Be patient above all else. Never criticize, correct, or scold Mom; always remember that Alzheimer's disease limits her abilities. Never take any resistance or agitation personally. It's not about your being right or winning; it is about her feeling safe, loved, comfortable, stimulated, and having fun.

Going a Little Deeper on the Magic Part: Creatively Stimulating, Loving, and Having Fun

I thought it might be helpful to provide more examples of what our remarkable caregivers did in helping Mom feel happier, be more stimulated, and have fun. Mom's caregivers were excellent at this. These actions are so important for brain health, emotional health, and happiness. I believe one of the key foundations of my mom's Alzheimer's longevity and happiness had everything to do with this magic. There are lots of ways for your caregivers to stimulate and have fun with your loved one with Dementia. Your loved one's fun and positive stimulation is only limited by your caregivers' time and imagination.

If your loved one lives in a facility that has talented, caring, loving, and creative caregivers and a good staff-to-patient ratio, then it is quite possible for your loved one to experience the same joy and longevity there that they would at home. Know that in a facility you may not be able to control whether the most talented, caring, and imaginative caregivers attend to your loved one, but I would ask for the caregivers that best connect with your loved one. If you don't see enough of these highly creative and loving caregivers, let your facility manager know you would like different caregivers, consider hiring a private caregiver of your choosing, or consider changing facilities.

Many facilities have planned activities for residents, and the more hours in your loved one's day dedicated to fun and connection, the happier and healthier your loved one will be. If your loved one is not engaged in fun and loving activities most of every day, then they probably are not stimulated and not enjoying themselves as much as they could and should be. As your loved one's disease progresses, it may be harder for your loved one to take advantage of group activities in a facility. It then will be important to make sure your loved one has a 1:1 caregiver most of the day to provide that stimulating and caring love and fun throughout their day; even very late in their dementia journey this is very important. Your list of activities to stimulate your loved one may be slightly different, but here is what really worked for Mom.

Art & Drawing

There are increasingly more studies showing that art is the type of cognitive stimulation that is good for brain and emotional health. It was great fun for Mom and built her self-esteem. The very favorite thing my mom loved to do was drawing in adult coloring books. Drawing with colored pencils helped Mom to focus, keep her mind active, relax, and feel content. I started out buying a couple of books at different craft stores and found colored pencils and crayons for her. She looked forward to it and really loved it. I noticed she liked using the pencils better than the crayons because the lines were more precise, and the overall drawing looked better and more professional. Ever since I can remember Mom liked doing things well and finishing projects. When Mom was drawing, she would smile. Her eyes would light up, and I knew she felt more confident, comfortable, and happy. These drawings, even very late in her journey, turned out beautifully. When they were complex and challenging, Mom dove right in, and patiently made them look great. She had a lot of pride in her work, which I'm sure gave her an important feeling of control and accomplishment. She exercised cognitive decision-making by choosing what colors and styles to use on each drawing. I know this activity was wonderful for her to be able to maintain hand-and-eye coordination, make decisions, and feel pride and a sense of accomplishment.

One time while I was sitting with Mom, I decided to add a few colors to her drawing creation. Though Mom had no words, she gently pushed my hand away from her drawing. Mom couldn't talk, but if I were to guess what she was thinking, it would have been, "You were never very good at drawing, Son; I love you, but you are really messing up my beautiful work!" Mom was prolific; I could not supply new books and colored pencils from the craft store fast enough. One of our wonderful caregivers suggested that we use Amazon as a place to find these adult coloring books. Luckily, they had what seemed like an endless supply of adult coloring books and pencils, which was necessary because Mom went through several books a week for years. Today, I cherish the many boxes of her completed coloring books. After that, Amazon became my Care Team's supply depot for many of Mom's projects, equipment, and medical supplies. They really helped me keep her happy and safe for many years. Having Amazon deliver everything Mom needed to our home gave me more confidence that I could take care of her at home, and because it was so easy, it gave me more time and energy to focus on Mom and our caregivers' needs. I saw Amazon as another critical member of Team Mom. Mom had great fun and enjoyment with her art, and her art was good for her, too.

Music

My mom loved listening to music especially all the oldies. She loved Frank Sinatra, Tony Bennet, Dinah Shore, the Big Bands, and many others. Our smart caregivers figured that out quickly and used their cell phones to play Mom's favorite music using Apple Music and other apps. This was a good, non-distracting, use of their cell phones. Mom would smile and bop her head at these familiar tunes. The caregiver would ask whether she liked a particular song or artist, and she would flash the most wonderful big smile and nod her head. I know music is also very good cognitive stimulation for a dementia patient. I know my mom was being stimulated and experiencing wonderful memories. For example, Mom and Dad were childhood sweethearts and both danced the Lindy together to many of these songs. When Mom heard the songs during her Alzheimer's journey, she would literally come alive physically and emotionally with love in her eyes, head bopping, and a big smile on her face. Mom had much fun as these songs stimulated her—and also relaxed her.

Magazines

Mom loved thumbing through fashion magazines with her caregivers. She would look at all the wonderful fashion photos and smile. The caregivers would point out different things about the magazine's models' clothing and ask Mom if she liked the dress or shoes. She would either nod yes or grimace and shake her head no. It was clear what she liked and did not like. This discernment was both fun and good for Mom cognitively. Picking up some fashion magazines at the local market and investing in a couple of subscriptions was well worth seeing Mom's big smile when she looked through these magazines.

Mom had always taken a lot of pride in how she dressed. When Mom was growing up, my grandmother was a seamstress in New York and would make beautiful dresses for her. My mom's friends from her old neighborhood in Brooklyn would tell Marina and me stories about how they would have to wait for Mom to iron her clothes before they went out. Mom still had that pride in how she looked every day throughout her entire Alzheimer's journey. These magazines fit right into her love of fashion and dressing nicely.

Your loved one may like magazines or books on different topics. The more pictures they have the better. Even late in their dementia journey, looking at magazines and pictures are a great way to stimulate your loved one cognitively, conjure memories and bring joy.

Daily Adventures

Mom loved to go on outings each day. Her wonderful caregivers would get her dressed, and they, with Marina or me, would take Mom out every day. I knew she loved going out because when she would use the walker going down the hall, she would excitedly point to the front door with a smile and a look of want on her face. We knew that meant "let's go out." We would take her to a grocery or other kind of store, a mall, or a park. We would also take her to a walkway above the beach and look at the ocean and scenery. Mom loved these daily adventures.

As a reminder, even though my mom walked with a walker around the house, for safety she used a wheelchair when we took her out for her daily adventure. Another benefit of the wheelchair was that she could see and experience more places more quickly without worrying about her falling. Mom especially enjoyed seeing children or pets on these outings. When a small child was near, she would light up with a big smile. The fact that mom taught kindergarten for so many years and loved children probably made these daily outings, when we saw children, even more delightful for her.

Her favorite place of all time to go to when she was out was the Sprinkles Ice Cream Store. I would get Mom a children's cup. She was so happy with her ice cream. A children's scoop, without nuts, was easy and safe to eat. Mom was so happy eating her ice cream. When she finished it, she would turn the cup upside down, pour every single drop onto her little spoon, and smile. Her concentration on getting every drop and her enjoyment were so cute and fun that I took a photo of her doing this and sent it to the head of marketing at Sprinkles. Sprinkles must have thought it was adorable, too, because they put the photo of Mom emptying every drop on their website. They told me they received so many wonderful responses to Mom's photo that they sent me a Sprinkles Gift Card and thank you card. The gift card of course was for free ice cream, which Mom loved.

Stimulating Play: Stuffed Animals, Dolls, and other Playtime Activities

Mom loved her stuffed animals and baby dolls. She would enjoy playing with them and hugging them. My wonderfully creative caregivers made up games to play with her and enjoyed many hours of delight with Mom and her dolls and stuffed animals. It was easy to see that playing with her dolls and stuffed animals was fun for Mom, but they were also very comforting to her. On the rare occasion when Mom was agitated and resisted what the caregiver wanted her to do, our clever creative caregivers used a doll or stuffed animal, which was a fun and comforting way to divert Mom's attention away from being agitated or resistant. Having Alzheimer's must be so scary, and anything that can be done to be comforting is a big plus. As I mentioned, attaching these same dolls and stuffed animals to Mom's walker and wheelchair made her feel warm and cared for.

Other Stimulating Activities

The above activities that Mom and her caregivers were involved in stimulated and delighted Mom. Other creative and stimulating activities she enjoyed were looking at photos, being read to, and puzzles. Mom also enjoyed watching Disney movies and many children's stories that were streaming on our TV. The Gilmore Girls was one of her favorite shows to watch because (I think) the show focused on a mother/daughter relationship. This show probably reminded her of the positive relationship she had with her mom and her daughter, my wonderful sister Marina.

Because television is not as stimulating and mentally engaging as many of these other activities, I encouraged our caregivers to limit Mom's TV time. It was okay for the TV to be in the background if Mom was also engaged in an activity that was more creative and interactive.

Much research shows that positive and fun stimulation is key for brain health. I'm not sure what your loved one will enjoy most, but I am sure you and your creative caregivers will figure out what is fun, stimulating, comforting. Think about and observe what your loved one likes. Whatever helps your loved one to be stimulated, experience less agitation, and feel loved is a very important part of a happier and potentially longer dementia journey. No one knows your loved one better than you and your dedicated remarkable caregivers.

Overall Thoughts on Caregiver Expectations

Really amazing caregivers perform well and naturally on all five of these top expectations. Even though I learned about most of these expectations from watching my best caregivers, create your own list based on your loved one's unique needs and wants. When you use your list for setting expectations, coaching, and recognizing and appreciating caregivers, you will be on your way to a happier and longer Alzheimer's journey with your loved one.

You may feel that this list is too detailed or too prescriptive. It may feel that way as you communicate it. However, remarkable caregivers want to be excellent and will appreciate your dedication to caregiving excellence and your mission for your loved one. I learned that each of these things were very important for Mom's breakthrough care. The most important thing is that you identify the expectations you have for your caregivers that lead to your loved one living longer and happier. Try to hold your care team to your high expectations and be clear with them. Like the coaching method, you are not being too formal or being a jerk communicating these specific expectations to your caregivers and then holding them accountable. You are being a loving care leader who wants the best for your loved one. When you hire high character, high capability, and highly responsive professional caregivers, they will appreciate what you are trying to do. They know what they are doing is part of a very important mission and a very noble purpose. They will not resist these expectations; they will appreciate knowing that you want the best for your loved one. Your remarkable caregivers will aspire to these expectations; ours did. Remember if you don't expect much, you won't get much.

Chapter Summary

1. The goal is to find and lead remarkable caregivers toward the mission of breakthrough results in longevity and joy for your loved one. As you watch the caregivers you have selected, you will

observe what great caregiving looks like and what is unacceptable to you. You will also see what your loved one reacts positively or negatively to.

2. As you watch and learn, you will develop your own list of caregiver expectations. It is likely to be very similar to this list but may be unique to your loved one's needs. Having your *Caregivers' Expectations List* will help you coach caregivers that may be very good but have an occasional lapse. The list will also help you recognize and reinforce the desired behaviors. Good is not good enough for breakthrough; your clear expectations, coaching, recognition, and reinforcement will take what are good caregivers and help them be remarkably great caregivers for your loved one.

3. To truly change the game and achieve breakthrough results, be sure your specific expectations list fall into two major categories:

    a. ***Safety Expectations:*** this area needs to be tailored to the unique physical and medical needs of your loved one.

    b. ***The Magic Expectations***: the areas of promoting fun, stimulation, familiarity, love, and comfort, or feeling safe. There are infinite ways your caregiver can bring this magic part of the breakthrough care to life.

CHAPTER 15

Retaining and Motivating Incredible Caregivers

An amazing and talented caregiver is a special gift for you and your loved one. We were blessed with some truly talented caregivers, but it did not happen by accident. First, I expanded the pool of talented caregivers to choose from by working with more than one agency. Then, I interviewed them with a proven interview method designed to know what they will be like on the job. Third, by recognizing what good and bad caregiving looked like, I learned how to use clear expectations, coaching, and recognition to help make very good caregivers even greater. I tried to learn something from each remarkable caregiver about what care actions seemed to work best for Mom. These continued insights became improvements on my list of Caregiving Expectations. I observed and learned about the important elements of keeping Mom safe and the magic subtleties of how caregivers creatively kept Mom stimulated, having fun, and feeling comforted and loved.

Once I was clearer on what I expected from Mom's caregivers and found an incredible caregiver it was critically important to retain and keep them motivated. As Mom's Alzheimer's progressed, I needed more of these remarkable caregivers for more shifts. Keeping each superpowered caregiver became everything. So, what did I learn about retaining and motivating these superstars? In my human resources career, I learned about motivating and retaining talent. I tried to apply these lessons to Team Mom. Here are some insights.

Pay Competitively

First, I tried to make sure my caregivers were paid competitively. I think people often underestimate how important this is. The caregivers for most of Mom's team for most of our journey came primarily from home care agencies. I found that the agencies that paid the most competitively had superior care talent. They must have believed in the saying employed by my ex-supervisor: "If you pay peanuts, you get squirrels" (no offense meant to any squirrels who are reading this book). A little better pay will help you find and keep a little better person. It is not the only factor, but it is a good beginning in the retention and motivation formula.

Flexibility in Shifts and Hours

After good pay, the next important factor is the shift and work flexibility needs of caregivers, who often have responsibilities for their own families. Being flexible around their family doctor appointments and other family commitments is worth a great deal to most caregivers. It was important for me to be flexible and meet all my highly talented caregivers' needs for desired workdays and hours. Also, when a caregiver had something important to do personally, working with several agencies made it much easier to find a substitute rather than refusing to grant the time off or having it be a problem. The fact that I was personally available to fill in for a caregiver if need be was also a big help.

As my small but powerful group of caregivers became a tight team, they would help each other by filling in for each other when needed. This was just one example of the great teamwork I saw among them. They all seemed to pull together for the higher purpose of helping Mom live longer and happier.

Because Mom needed supervision around the clock during her later years, all five of our caregivers worked full time for Mom, and each were given the exact days and shifts that they wanted. Some of our caregivers preferred nighttime, others preferred days. Some liked weekends, some weekdays, Overall, I tried to keep their shifts to around eight hours and about 40 hours per week. Not working longer than eight hours a day and

40 hours a week ensured everyone was alert, focused, and motivated to provide the best possible care for Mom. Working much more than eight hours a day in a short time brings fatigue, irritability, burn-out, and lack of attention. You don't want any of that for your loved one. I wanted each of their A+ game for every second of every shift. Also, the result of each caregiver having their desired shift and hours is that Mom became the only person they cared for. This is a big advantage, first because our caregivers felt loyal and stayed with Mom, and second, they were able to be super focused on knowing Mom better. Finally, had they worked for more clients, they could have introduced a virus or bacteria that might have put Mom's health at greater risk.

Engagement

When you find high-achieving caregivers who have compassion and creativity, they want to be actively engaged in the mission. When the mission is noble and clear and your expectations for excellent caregiving are clear, your remarkable caregivers will be like one of those wind-up toys that you point in the right direction and off they go because they will be excited and clear about what they are doing! This is especially true in the "create magic" part of your expectations, where they get to tap into their creative superpowers to creatively have fun, stimulate, engage, and comfort your loved one. When they feel supported by you, the care leader, and trust you, you will be amazed by what they can and will do for you and your precious loved one.

Recognition and Appreciation

Drawing again from my human resources experience, recognition and appreciation is very important for anyone. Taco Bell and their parent YUM! Brands created an outstanding culture of recognition and appreciation. All leaders were asked to create their own personal recognition award. Leaders were encouraged to pick a personal recognition award that reflected who you were, the type of work you did, and the behaviors or results important for the success of your department or function. My award was called the People Grower Award. I recognized people that demonstrated great people growing skills; for my People Grower recognition award I gave each person a small bag of seeds, a trowel, and a plaque describing what they did to grow their people. There were hundreds of these leaders' personal recognition awards across all the YUM! Brands companies. These personal recognition rewards did a wonderful job in reinforcing an employee's performance while at the same time reinforcing the desired behaviors and the culture overall. It was also fun and creative for the people who gave them and fun and reinforcing for people who received them.

My caregivers were very important to me, so drawing from these insights about the importance of recognizing greatness, I did my best to recognize great work and the right behaviors of each member of my little caregiving team. My goal was to help each person on Team Mom feel appreciated, respected, highly valued, and a part of the family. When I saw one of my caregivers do something creative in entertaining and stimulating Mom, I would tell them what a great idea it was and how lucky I was to have them on Team Mom. I also would share their great idea with the rest of the care team. Also, when we were out with Mom at the Sprinkles Ice Cream Store or another fun destination, I would often get our caregivers a little gift or treat as another small way for them to feel appreciated and valued. I would be sure to celebrate birthdays, holidays, and other important events in their life. Mom was so happy and loved these celebrations and little parties. Marina and I also would really get to know each caregiver personally and we wanted them to get to know us too. This special bond we had with each caregiver lasted; we still celebrate with most of our caregivers today.

Our remarkable caregivers not only helped Marina and me take care of Mom, but each has helped us personally. They all knew we appreciated them, and they comforted and encouraged us, too. Seeing our loved one experience this long steady decline is, as you may already know, very emotionally difficult and exhausting. Occasionally when I felt down or discouraged as care leader, having such wonderful, caring, and fun caregivers was therapeutic for me and my sister as well. They all had been through this journey with other patients and families and some even with their own families. They knew what Marina and I were going through, and they knew just what to do or say to help us when we needed it. Appreciation, recognition, and feeling belonging are powerfully motivating. Sincerely appreciating someone does not cost anything and can be huge in keeping a wonderful care team. My wise Sicilian Grandfather used to say, "for the same money, you can be nice to people." He was right, appreciating others is so simple and yet is so powerful.

These retention and motivation actions really work. Some members of Team Mom were with us longer than others, but the shortest tenure among our five wonderful and talented caregivers was three years. Three of the five caregivers were with us from the very beginning when I started needing help with Mom's care. Finding, then keeping, and motivating your great care team is critical for breakthrough care results. These approaches are simple. Pay better than most places, use multiple agencies to provide the greatest flexibility to meet everyone's unique shift needs, and then make them feel recognized, appreciated, and an important part of the family. These retention and motivation strategies were essential to keeping our superpowered caregivers for a very long time and essential to our mission of Mom living longer and happier. Finding them and then doing everything possible to keep remarkable caregivers who keep your loved one safe, stimulated, comforted, and loved is very doable. Don't forget my Sicilian grandmother's "If it's been done before, you can do it, too."

Chapter Summary

1. When you work to find incredible caregivers, you also want to work hard to motivate and retain them. If a caregiver is amazing, the longer this incredible caregiver stays with your loved one the better. Because they know each other so well, you loved one will feel comfortable with them and fulfilled by them which

increases your loved one's likelihood of being safer, happier, and living longer.

2. When you or your agency pays well, you will have a bigger pool of the most talented caregivers. This increases your chances of finding and keeping the best of the best caregivers.

3. Don't underestimate the real power of being flexible and creative in meeting your care team's needs and wants for certain work hours, days, and shifts. Working the shift and days someone wants is an underrated powerful motivation and retention tool.

4. Be cautious about shifts that are too long. Truly excellent caregiving is mentally and physically demanding. A caregiver can lose focus and energy if they work too long a shift or too many days in a row. This can negatively impact their focus on safety, fun, stimulation, and affection for your loved one. Try to limit shifts to no more than eight hours and 40 hours a week.

5. Recognition, appreciation, and respect are huge factors that motivate and retain incredible caregivers. Everyone likes to be recognized and appreciated for who they are and what they do. These things cost nothing but pay big dividends. Be creative, thoughtful, and personal in recognizing and appreciating your wonderful caregivers. It can be as simple as sincerely saying "thank you" and "you are doing such a great job".

CHAPTER 16

Visualizing Great Care Helps Achieve Great Care

If you have a picture in your mind of what amazing caregiving looks like, then you are much more likely to know what you are looking for. I found it helpful to have a picture in my mind of an amazing caregiver. If your vision of great caregiving is clear in your mind, you will know great caregiving when you see it with your loved one.

To visualize what great caregiving looks like, you might find this snapshot of our remarkable caregivers as one example or picture of what great caregiving can look like. Helped in part by my sourcing, selection, evaluation, retention, and motivation work, I was blessed with truly great caregivers who took beautiful care of Mom for a very long time.

Each gifted caregiver was special in their own way. They all met and exceeded my high standards of safety, fun, stimulation, caring, and love for Mom. Four of the five amazing caregivers were experienced and licensed CNAs (Certified Nursing Assistants); and another became an RN (Registered Nurse) while she was working with my mom. It was my job as care leader to create an environment that brought out the very best of each of their creative and compassionate special talents. Each of these amazing ladies contributed in large ways to Mom's longevity and happiness.

Sylvia

Sylvia was the first caregiver whom I hired. She ended up staying with my mom the entire time. Sylvia pursued her RN Nursing Degree during the time she was with Mom. Even though she was going to school at the same time, I never once felt she was distracted with the things going on with her personal life or with school. It was the opposite; she brought her nursing learning to Mom. During our journey with Sylvia, she got engaged, married, and had a child. During her wedding planning time, I recall Sylvia sharing with Mom many photos of her wedding dress and other aspects of wedding planning. Mom lit up and smiled when she looked at all the pictures. When Marina and I showed Sylvia Mom's wedding photos, she and Mom both beamed with joy. In all the pictures, I could see how beautiful Mom's dress, made by my grandmother, was. I could also see how happy Mom was. The entire event looked amazing. I'm sure Sylvia picked up a few pointers from those photos for her wedding.

Because Sylvia worked for her grandmother, who ran a board and care home, she knew a lot about caregiving. Combining this with her nursing studies, Sylvia knew what supplies were needed supplies and what medical issues a patient with dementia experiences. For example, Sylvia told me about special hip pads that would cushion Mom's hips if she ever fell. Sylvia's extensive wound care knowledge was helpful in getting the right type of ointment and pads to make sure Mom never got bed sores or other skin irritations and wounds. She really knew safety and other products that really helped Mom stay safe and comfortable at home over a very long period. Sylvia was the caregiver who introduced me to Amazon as a resource for medical supplies, adult coloring books, and many other things Mom needed during her Alzheimer's journey.

Sylvia told me once that she could not work for us any longer because she was not happy with something her home care agency was doing and wanted to change to a different agency. I told her I would switch to any agency she wanted because I did not want to lose her. Wanting to keep Sylvia, I quickly contracted with Sylvia's new agency. I was thereby able to keep Sylvia and because, by doing this, I demonstrated my loyalty to her, she felt even greater loyalty to us. An agency is important but not nearly as important as retaining an incredible, loyal, and talented, long-time caregiver. After Sylvia got married, she moved over an hour away, but she did the long commute and still reliably and lovingly took care of Mom on a regular basis.

My mom and Sylvia had many fun times and really loved each other. Sylvia was compassionate and creative in her care of Mom. She also was highly sensitive and tuned into Mom's environment and what she needed to be safer and make Mom's life more enjoyable. She would often ask me if we could get this or that for Mom. I appreciated her initiative and gladly did. It was a pleasure supporting Sylvia because she brought compassion, skill, and creativity to her work. Sylvia is now a wonderful and loving stay-at-home mom with two beautiful children. Bless you, Sylvia, and thank you for all your wonderful care, the medical knowledge you generously shared, and the love you gave Mom for so many years.

Paula

Paula is also one of the first caregivers I hired; she also stayed with Mom for the entire journey. Paula is one of the most thoughtful, caring, and creative people I have ever had the pleasure of knowing. On the surface, she is quiet and reserved, but she had a tenacity and real passion when caring for Mom. Paula brought a quiet sensitivity plus a wonderful sense of humor and creativity to the team. Paula also was an incredibly compassionate and caring listener to Mom as well as to Marina and me. She and my mom had a wonderful connection, filled with magic and trust when they were together, and Mom's eyes twinkled when they were together. They did not have to be *doing* much to have great fun. As a son, watching them interact so beautifully gave me great happiness and comfort. Paula would always give Mom the feeling of great joy. Paula was the first to play Mom's favorite music. She also was the first to try the coloring books that Mom enjoyed and loved so much. Clearly, Paula and Mom really loved and appreciated each other. The longer Paula was with us, the more their love and affection grew for each other. Paula also had a very strong connection with my sister Marina, becoming a terrific listener and friend to her as we struggled emotionally through Mom's journey.

Since Paula liked to work the day shift during the weekdays, she was the caregiver who helped take Mom out the most. She did a great job in our fun outings, and she helped make all Mom's doctor appointments smooth and fun. (I will talk more about what I learned about working with our doctor care team in Chapters 20 and 21.)

Paula managed to make doctor visits fun for Mom by entertaining her while we waited for the doctor. Paula would entertain me, too. We would make fun bets on how long it would take to see the doctor and on how long the doctor would spend with us. Don't worry, neither Paula nor I have a gambling problem! Anyone who has been to a doctor knows this time ratio is sometimes not good. Most people spend a lot longer waiting for the doctor than the doctor spends with them. Paula would start the iPhone timer when we sat down in the waiting room. Paula always won the bet on how long it would take to get to see the Doctor (I guess I was too optimistic). I won the bet on how long the Doctor would spend with us. Don't tell Paula, but I cheated on the latter; I would choose a longer time than Paula, and to help ensure I won, if the doctor was speeding, I would quietly ask him a few more questions from my doctors' list of questions (see Chapter 21). This helped me win the bet and helped us because the doctor took more time with Mom.

I know that dementia patients can become agitated if they must wait too long in the waiting room. Mom never became agitated because Paula was an expert at keeping her entertained, occupied, and respectful of others waiting to see the doctor. She quietly teased Mom to make her laugh or comforted her by gently massaging her arm. She also brought coloring books or magazines for them to look at together.

Like Sylvia, Paula has a quiet yet very strong faith that I have seen her rely on and which I'm sure strengthened her ability to be an amazing caregiver. My sister and I are still very good friends with Paula, who has been a great blessing to us for a very long time. Thank you, Paula, for your great care ideas and your wonderful help to Mom, Marina, and me.

Amanda

I brought on Amanda near the beginning, too. Despite being a little older than our other caregivers, Amanda has so much energy, strength, and life in her that she inspired the whole team. Originally from Peru, Amanda entered the house with positive and fun Peruvian energy that always lit up the place. She would jokingly say that she had all this energy because she had "llama power."

When Amanda arrived for her night shifts and Sunday day shift, she and Mom hugged, and Mom would give her a big kiss on the cheek. It was comforting for me to see that Mom was so happy and in a great mood after her time with Amanda. Amanda exhibited much love, caring, and creativity in caring for Mom. Like all members of Team Mom, when there was a shift change, I always noticed each caregiver was highly professional and really cared about Mom's well-being. When a caregiver arrived for a shift, she would immediately ask the departing caregiver how Mom was feeling and if there was anything bothering her or anything they should watch for in the upcoming shift. I was happy they were a real team and that they coordinated so well with each other. All the caregivers being bilingual, Luisa started a shift change habit of lovingly saying "hello jefe (boss)! How is jefa del jefe?" If I were the boss, they knew Mom was the Chairman of the Board. They were right!

One example of Amanda's amazing professionalism and commitment to Mom occurred on one of her overnight shifts. She was helping Mom get out of bed one night, and their legs got a little tangled up. Mom started to fall. Rather than letting Mom fall to the ground, Amanda pulled Mom toward herself, guiding Mom to lean against her instead of falling to the floor. Amanda ended up twisting her ankle; Mom was completely fine. I could see that Amanda acted selflessly and cared enough to prevent a possible Mom fall. I find it a heroic act that Amanda would rather get hurt herself than risk Mom getting hurt. I felt so grateful to have such wonderful caregivers. In a couple of weeks, Amanda's ankle healed. Other members of Team Mom gladly helped by filling in for her while she was out. We were truly a proud team of caregivers that helped each other to help Mom.

Marina and I still see Amanda regularly. She still has her amazing Peruvian llama power and her kindness, energy, and zest for life. When we see Amanda these days, we like to give her little llama mementos of appreciation. Like all our caregivers, Amanda is an amazingly beautiful person who has helped us significantly as we traveled Mom's Alzheimer's journey together. Bless you, Amanda, and thank you so much for sharing your llama energy with us.

Luisa

Luisa came to us a little later in Mom's journey and was another remarkable member of Team Mom. Luisa was also always positive and compassionate with Mom. Whenever Luisa walked into our home and saw my mom, she would give Mom a big hug and a kiss on the cheek and loudly and enthusiastically say. "Hello, Principessa!!" Mom would then share a big smile, and her face would beam with happiness. Luisa would then turn to me and energetically say, "Hello, Jefe!" Luisa always brightened the room; joyous is the only way I can describe Luisa. Some people have a special gift that clearly shows how much they love life and caring for others. Like all our amazing caregivers, Luisa has a very strong personal faith, and you can see that in all aspects of her life. Touch is very important to all of us, and I believe it is especially important to many Alzheimer's patients and was to Mom in particular. All our caregivers were very loving to Mom and would often hug her, hold her hand, or kiss her cheek. Luisa was the most expressive care member of our team, and Mom responded very positively to her. Even though Mom could not speak, you could see what a compassionate listener Luisa was with Mom; she would show so much compassion and caring for Mom. You could see Mom's happiness as she felt completely understood by her. Luisa had abounding creative energy for having fun with Mom and lifting her spirits.

Luisa believed strongly in eating natural and healthy foods, which reinforced the power of good nutrition for Mom. She introduced me to the NutriBullet Personal Blender and how natural smoothies and soups are not only easy to prepare but would be great for Mom's health. When Mom was hospitalized later in her journey and I was staying with her, Luisa brought me homemade healthy soups and shakes with compelling, positive energy, saying, "Drink this; you have to stay strong for Mamasita!!" Her kind of positivity and love made a huge difference and helped my sister and me be strong for Mom.

Luisa and Mom had many wonderful and fun times together. Luisa would sing to her, sometimes in Spanish, and Mom would smile and shake her hips like she was dancing. Luisa sometimes worked overnight and when Mom had trouble sleeping, I sometimes could hear the two of them laughing and having a great time. One overnight shift when Luisa and Mom were a little too noisy, Luisa told me that Mom cutely pointed to my room next door, then to her lips, and made a "ssshhh" gesture, meaning "Ssshh! Let's not wake up Mark; he needs his sleep!!" I found this cute and heartwarming: Mom, even with her Alzheimer's, wanted to take care of me.

Sometimes, I would hear Luisa lovingly tell Mom "God loves you, and thinks you are so special." Mom would smile and nod her head. Luisa would also say cute prayers and sing little songs to Mom. Mom savored these precious moments. She adored and responded to Luisa and all five of her superstar caregivers with love and enjoyment. Bless you Luisa, you are truly extraordinary and took such beautiful care of our "Principessa."

Alma

Finally, Alma was the most recent addition to Team Mom. She was very sweet, creative, and compassionate with my mom, too. Alma was with us for only three years, but like the others, she had a special way to keep Mom happy and calm. Like the others as well, she believed in the healing power of touch and would always give Mom a special kiss on her cheek and wonderful bear hugs, clearly comforting and calming her. Mom treasured Alma, and Alma loved Mom. Although Mom could not speak at all, the two of them communicated without words in amazing ways. Quieter than our other caregivers, Alma nonetheless made Mom smile. Mom appeared calm, happy, and secure with Alma, obviously feeling supported and understood. Sometimes, the two of them would make funny faces in the mirror together until they both laughed, and so did I when I saw this. They understood each other very well and communicated in the most delightful way. Alma was amazing at knowing exactly what Mom wanted. There weren't any words between them, just wonderfully funny faces, but Alma knew what Mom was thinking. The joy that they shared was magical.

I felt Mom was very safe with all our incredible caregivers. With Alma, though, there was something extra; she had a laser focus on Mom's safety and anticipated what Mom was going to do long before she did anything. Her keen observation skills and insights ensured Mom was extra safe especially when she was standing or walking with the walker. Alma always put her arms around my mom, and Mom always kept her hands on the walker when they walked down the hallway together. When Mom was transitioning from the toilet, bed, or chair to a standing position, Alma paid close attention to where Mom's feet were and where her own feet were so there was no chance of a fall. Alma was laser-focused and diligent about fall prevention. I felt great confidence that, with every transition, Mom was ultra-safe with Alma. When Mom ate her meals, Alma was also laser-focused on how much food my mom put in her mouth, how small the pieces were, and how Mom was swallowing her food or liquid. She would watch Mom's throat like a hawk to confirm she was ready to take another bite of food or to take another drink of liquid before she allowed her to put more in her mouth. Alma knew how easy it is for Alzheimer's patients to choke or aspirate fluid or food into their lungs and was careful to ensure it didn't happen. Alma was really on top of all aspects of her game, especially when it came to mom's safety.

Alma and Mom would quietly have fun teasing each other about their coloring book drawings, and both would quietly point in fun ways to the drawings they had made. Mom and Alma enjoyed a great friendship and treasured being with each other. Alma completed our incredible and powerful award-winning caregiving team. Bless Alma as she kept Mom super safe, calm, and entertained on her journey.

Marina

Marina is not a caregiver as you are already aware. She is my sister. By including my sister, you will see some of the other important roles that family members or even friends can play on your care team.

I am a huge NBA Basketball fan, and, in the NBA, there is an award called "Sixth Man of the Year." Five players play on the floor at any one time. Our five caregivers were Mom's Championship Care Team. Basketball fans know that no team wins NBA Championship without an amazing sixth man on their team; when that player comes on the floor, he lifts the team to new heights. The sixth man on our championship team was Marina, who did loads to lift and bolster Team Mom.

Marina did the washing and cleaning so that our caregivers could exclusively focus on providing those breakthrough experiences for Mom. Alzheimer's patients, especially later in their journey, can become incontinent and create a lot of laundry. Marina not only did washing, cleaning, and helping in the yard, but she also helped me cook many healthy meals for Mom. All Marina's efforts enabled our caregivers to focus completely on Mom to provide that magic connection that helped Mom be happy and safe. Marina's help also allowed me to focus on being a good care leader and have the time to work on improving all the aspects of breakthrough care.

Marina and Mom had a lot of fun together and I saw how much they loved each other and enjoyed being together. Marina brought happiness and love to Mom's life and inspired the caregivers to do the same. She worked closely with the caregivers, too, and was a wonderful sounding board for me and all the many care-leader decisions to be made. Marina was not only our championship Sixth Man of the Year but also my Assistant Team Manager, Facility Manager, and Team Cheerleader. Team Mom would not have won the longevity and happiness championship without Marina.

Visualizing Success: The Common Traits of Remarkable Caregiving

I wanted you to get to know our caregiver team a little and how special they were so you can get a small picture in your mind of great caregiving. My hope is that this helps you keep your standards very high as you evaluate caregivers for your loved one. Finding a superpowered care team is possible with high standards and clear expectations, multiple agency sourcing, great selection interviewing, thoughtful coaching, and evaluation, as well as solid retention and motivation strategies.

Incredible care givers can look a little different from each other and yet they are powerfully the same in many other ways. I found with our caregiver team each of their personalities and how they expressed their skills to be different; yet, they also had very important common skills, backgrounds, and common strengths. Knowing these common traits will help you know what to look for as you source and evaluate caregivers for your special loved one. These are the common traits I noticed in all our superpowered caregivers:

The Common Traits of Remarkable Caregivers

1. They all had great pride and joy in their work; they each knew how important their work was to Mom, to Marina, and to me. Most important, taking care of Mom was clearly significant and motivating to each of them.

2. They all had at least a couple of years of Dementia Care experience and at minimum a CNA (Certified Nursing Assistant) Certification.

3. Each, in a different way, all seemed to derive great love, caring and strength from their belief system, their faith, and the importance of family.

4. They all had a great, positive sense of humor that brought joy to their work. They took their work seriously but not themselves.

5. They brought their "A" game to every hour of every shift. I never saw anyone just "putting in the hours." They brought professionalism, creativity, empathy, compassionate energy, and personality to Mom consistently all the time. Their passion and enthusiasm to keep Mom safe and happy was infectious. In every way, they truly wanted to show Mom how much they loved and cared for her and wanted Mom to feel joyous, safe, secure, and to have fun.

6. They each were open to feedback and learning new things. They all had excellent basic skills and experience but also worked on improving their knowledge and ability.

7. They knew and loved their mission to help Mom live longer and happier. They were focused on Mom and knew my priorities. They lived every moment of every shift to help make Mom's journey fun, stimulating, warm, familiar, and most of all safe. They exuded creativity, compassion, love, and patience, and Mom always felt like she was special and their priority no matter what was happening in their own lives.

Chapter Summary

1. You as care leader will see glimpses of many of these powerful and positive traits as you interview caregivers and when they work their first shift or two. Make sure you are watchful in the beginning so you can notice these powerful traits (or not).

2. Basic Safety skills should be similar and strong across your caregiving team. The chapters in this book on safety practices are designed to make sure you know what safe caregiving looks like. However, how your caregivers brings fun, comfort, creativity, stimulation, and love to your loved may differ and reflect each of their special and unique qualities. This is normal and good. If you see a great idea on how one caregiver connects beautifully with your loved one, as care leader share these great ideas with

others on your care team. Sharing good ideas from one caregiver across your team is recognition and will build the self-esteem and loyalty as they see the importance of their ideas or practices you shared.

3. If you find one of these remarkable caregivers with these special traits, do everything in your power to make sure they stay with your loved one for as long as possible. It is important to work hard at meeting the needs of these incredible caregivers. The longer your remarkable caregivers spend time with your loved one, the better off your loved one will be. It is well worth your effort as care leader to use some of the tactics in the last chapter to keep and motivate these incredibly special caregivers.

4. Do not settle!!! Like any worker, there are poor, average, and remarkable caregivers. Be accountable as care leader to find and keep remarkable caregivers! You and your loved one will be very happy you did!

I was so blessed and am so grateful that I had such a wonderful group of caregivers to love and take care of Mom. They were amazing in so many ways. They gave me peace of mind with Mom and supported my sister and me wonderfully. I share who they are and their common traits so that you, too, can find such caregivers and experience the joy that I did in having a wonderful team of helpers for your loved one. If you can keep amazing caregivers for a long time, they will go a long way to implementing the components of breakthrough care, helping your loved one live longer and happier.

Your life will be better with these great caregivers, too. I am confident you can use your care leader superpowers to find them, retain them, and for a very long time keep them motivated and focused on your loved one.

CHAPTER 17

A Final Thought on The Gift of Superhero Caregivers

Amazing caregivers ensure essential safety for your loved one and help keep them mobile, active, and engaged. They also bring your loved one familiarity, fun, comfort, cognitive stimulation, and feeling loved. They ensure your loved one eats safely and healthily and takes their medicines, vitamins, and supplements to help them with their cognitive and physical health. Team Mom caregivers were extremely sensitive and observant of Mom and knew her so well that they would alert me if they observed something slightly off or medically wrong with Mom. I could then get Mom to the doctor quickly if necessary. Their knowledge of Mom and their highly tuned skills of observation were key in identifying medical issues early enough to avoid more serious medical problems later. They ensured Mom was safe 24 hours a day and made certain that she was engaged, stimulated, happy, and loved during her entire Alzheimer's Journey. Each caregiver, in her unique way, brought the gift of joy to Mom. Some facilities, for many reasons, don't have the coverage necessary to ensure your loved one is enriched and safe every minute of their day. Private caregiver superstars can fill this gap and help ease your worries, too. Great caregivers will love and care for your loved one and bring you great peace of mind and even provide some emotional care for you as well.

As Mom's long-term care leader, with a little help from my HR corporate experience, I learned a great deal about finding, selecting, retaining, and motivating a group of incredible caregivers. The most important insight is that you as care leader are the key to making all this work. If you have the passion for your loved one, you can learn about great caregiving and finding and keeping these superstars. It starts with your empowered love and passion for your loved one.

The tools and methods in this Leader's Playbook are the bridge between your passion and your loved one's longer and happier life. When you see your amazing caregivers do what they do best, your vision and expectations will become clearer. As you visualize greatness, you can recognize each caregiver who exemplifies these high expectations and coach those who miss something on occasion. Your care leadership will then become a virtuous cycle; you will find and motivate great caregivers, which will bring you greater clarity of success; this success will raise your standards and motivate you to support your caregivers to create greater breakthrough care and a longer happier life for your loved one. You will know you are doing amazing things to help your loved one, and you will feel even better about yourself. Team Mom was a true gift that I know you can have for your loved one and yourself too!

Leading Physicians & Other Specialists on Your Team

CHAPTER 18

Overview

Physicians and other specialists are also critical members of your loved one's team. As part of Team Mom, I had very high expectations of all these specialists, too. Having the mindset that these very independent specialists worked for me and for Mom helped me be a better leader of them for Mom's care. I think some doctors may not act as if they work for their patients or their families, but the best ones were fine with my high expectations for their time, answering my questions, and being highly accountable to us. It was important that each doctor bring their A+ game for Mom. I noticed that when I was acting as a bold care leader and expected a lot from them, I would get better information from the physicians, and they would take better care of Mom. Upon occasion a physician could be a little pretentious, which can get in the way of compassion and care. It is important to be a strong care leader and not allow yourself to be rushed or bullied by physicians or anyone else when it comes to your loved one's care. Mom needed and deserved the best care on the planet, regardless of anyone's ego or schedule. I had to make sure they were taking enough time and showing enough compassion, care, and creativity to be worthy enough to be on Mom's care team.

Often, a physician, due to ego, may be reluctant to consider opposing information or have their judgement questioned in any way. As a good care leader and advocate your role is to treat high-ego physicians as having a valued point of view but not treat anything they say as *ex cathedra* or infallible. It may help to reframe a physician's perceived self-importance as a weakness because it usually is. Too much ego and lack of openness to opposing points of view can limit their mindset and their ability to learn, be creative, and improve as a physician. Physicians are key to your loved one living longer and happier, but it is important that you manage them, too.

CHAPTER 19

Building Enough
Medical Knowledge

When I was in human resources, I had a team of specialists working for me. Some had deeper knowledge than I had in certain areas, but I had enough knowledge to guide them. Leading your loved one's physician team is similar. You won't know as much as a physician about medicine, but you can learn enough to communicate with them and to provide excellent leadership, advocacy, and decision making for your loved one.

To play this role it is important to have basic medical knowledge about your loved one's medical condition(s) and the associated implications. Learning about Mom's medical conditions, possible treatments and potential tradeoffs was very helpful to me as Mom's care leader. I developed a foundation of knowledge so I could ask good questions and make better decisions about any of her doctors' suggested treatments.

The best way I have found to get started building this important knowledge is to search the best medical websites. Occasionally I would go deeper to read some of the research referenced in these medical websites or even read a book on a medical topic. The general medical website that I liked the best as a starting point is *mayoclinic.org*. Several doctors recommended this site to me. Large reputable medical universities are also good places to learn. Specifically, I also rely on *pubmed.ncbi*, *clevelandclinic.org* and *health.harvard.edu*. The resources section of this book lists more sources of reliable medical information. Don't be intimidated by the medical language in these studies. If you encounter a term or word you don't know, just google it, or look it up in the search bar of these medical websites. I have no formal medical training, and I was still able to understand the research reports' findings.

After doing some basic research, then compare what you've learned online against information from your loved one's doctor or other trusted doctors with whom you confer. Remember that your loved one's condition may differ somewhat from the general condition you read about. It is very good to compare information across sources. The more you know the better you will be able to be a knowledgeable advocate and decision maker for your loved one. Dementia and Alzheimer's patients usually cannot be their own advocate or decision maker.

If your loved one is in a facility, don't just assume that the facility will manage your loved one's medical care effectively. Be proactive, and be close enough to your loved one's health to know their medical needs and learn about their medical conditions so you can be an effective advocate and decision maker. If you wait for the facility to tell you about your loved one's medical problems, it may be too late to avoid a potentially dangerous hospital visit.

Chapter Summary

1. A loved one with dementia needs an advocate and decision maker. Having a foundation of medical knowledge for the medical conditions your loved one has is necessary for good advocacy and good decision making.

2. There are many ways to build know-how about your loved one's conditions. These include reputable general medical websites such as mayoclinic.org as well as research universities' specialized medical websites and associated published studies. You can also talk with other specialist doctors you respect. Having more than one source of information provides the necessary checks and balances for your loved one's care.

3. Don't be intimidated by the technical nature of some medical studies. You don't have to be a medical professional to have an

opinion and pose good questions to your loved one's doctor. If you triangulate your sources by getting information from a couple different places, your medical knowledge and insights can be even more reliable, and you will be pleasantly surprised how much you can learn in a short amount of time.

CHAPTER 20

Physicians and Medical Gurus: The Prescription for Breakthrough

Neurologist

The neurologist specializing in dementia care is one of the most important members of your care team. An expert at diagnosing the specific kind of dementia that your loved one has, this type of doctor can tell you about the nuances of various types of dementias, the stage your loved one is in, and the specific behaviors and medical issues to expect at each stage. We were fortunate to have one of the leading dementia centers in the country, UC Irvine Institute for Memory Impairments and Neurological Disorders (UCI MIND), in Irvine, not far from us. We went there for Mom's initial diagnosis; given the high quality and reputation of the center, we stayed with UCI MIND for neurology expertise and regular clinical care throughout Mom's journey.

We loved our UCI MIND neurologist, Dr. Aimee Pierce. Her insights on Mom's Alzheimer's and the associated behaviors were excellent. She also was outstanding at understanding how Mom's other medical conditions and symptoms as well as her other medicines affected and might affect her Alzheimer's. Because great neurology advice was so important to mom, Mom also had a second neurologist, Dr. Teryn Clarke, who I would compare advice with. She, too, was amazing and wonderful. I wanted to be sure all the neurology recommendations were confirmed and aligned between sources. These two wonderful women often had a slightly different spin on mom's brain care, but the fundamentals of their advice were aligned. They both openly shared with us the likely impact of various medicines, other doctors' recommended treatments, and other things affecting Mom's dementia. We greatly appreciated them; they were immensely helpful to us.

As mentioned, Mom's original diagnosis and the prognosis of Mom living only five more years from Dr. Pierce drove me to try all these many small actions that ended up being game changing for Mom. In retrospect, I am grateful for her directness in this. The Kennedy family mantra,[1] "when the going gets tough, the tough get going," rang in my ears. Mom did live nearly three times longer than our wonderful neurologist predicted on that scary prognosis day. I am confident that Mom would have lived even longer had a physician not made a tragic medical error toward the end of her life (more on this in Chapter 25).

A word on prognoses: they are based on statistics, experience, and averages It is important to know that when a doctor shares with you a likely result, side effect, or prognosis, they draw from their personal experience and from results of medical studies. Even if a physician tries to be objective, his or her experience will be influenced by lived experience or study. Also, a physician's insight from a study can be influenced by demographic bias or be an average result. Your loved one is unique and special, and their medical situation will not fit into an average. This does not mean you shouldn't listen closely to your doctor's ideas and suggestions. However, be sure to ask knowledge-based questions to help filter out potential biases and bring the best information and your loved one's uniqueness to medical decisions for your loved one.

Many people rely on their Primary Care Physician to be the only doctor their loved one sees for basic dementia care. The PCP is a very important player on your team, but I found the neurologists on Team Mom were the experts on Alzheimer's and therefore much more able to guide us on all aspects of her Alzheimer's.

---

1. Most famously used by Joseph Kennedy, father of JFK, RKF, and their siblings, to motivate their family (OUP, 2025), the phrase, known as an *antimetabole*—a rhetorical device where words are repeated in reverse order for emphasis, has been attributed to many people over the years and has now become a common phrase.

Primary Care Physician

An outstanding PCP is also a critical member of your care team. Elderly loved ones overall, and especially those with dementia, are predisposed to many medical problems. Some of these problems are linked to dementia, and others are a part of normal aging. Because of these problems, it was important for me to have regular and quick access to Mom's primary doctor. Dr. Ahuja was Mom's PCP, and she was excellent.

One example of the benefits of an accessible PCP is that Mom would occasionally have trouble with her delicate skin. Sometimes, she would have the beginning of a routine rash, sore, or a scrape. After a brief description on the phone, Dr. Ahuja would simply call in an antibiotic or anti-fungal ointment for treatment. You shouldn't have to experience the challenge of taking a late-stage dementia patient into a specialist's office for something very routine for your loved one. Of course, for more complex issues or issues that don't get easily resolved, it is a good idea to have a specialist like a dermatologist available as part of your extended care team. Mom's guru dermatologist, Dr. Worswick was terrific. He was a leader in his field and practiced at USC Keck Medicine. He knew the difficulty of coming in to see him, so he would often simply ask that we send a photo of Mom's skin condition, and then he would call in the appropriate prescription. Being a medical guru, he was always spot on with his diagnosis and treatment.

I found Mom's Dr. Ahuja willing to speak to me over the phone about Mom's issues without hesitation. Easy phone access to the doctor was very important in determining what we should do to help Mom in certain situations. If your loved one's doctor is one of those doctors who always insists you come into the office even if it is for something routine, or you can't get an appointment with them within 48 hours, it may be time for a new PCP for your team. You should not be forced to go to urgent care for everything short term. In the same way you shouldn't settle for a poor or average caregiver, you shouldn't settle for an average or poor PCP. An inaccessible PCP who will not readily talk to you on the phone is a poor doctor. Because of the nature of what a PCP treats, a dementia patient needs quick and easy access to the PCP. There are plenty of very good physicians to choose from. Everyone on your care team needs to be highly accessible and excellent. Your loved one deserves the best, and so do you.

Dr. Ahuja prescribed most of Mom's regular medications, like her blood pressure, thyroid, and cholesterol medicines. Given the accessibility of Mom's PCP, I had her handle our refills for her Alzheimer's prescriptions for Aricept and Namenda. That way, she was also aware of the prescriptions of Mom's other medical specialists, helping avoid interaction side effects. Mom's PCP was a good care integrator and helped me liaison across specialties because I found a few doctors surprisingly either don't know that much about side effects or don't like to talk about side effects and drug interactions. To be extra certain, I also consulted regularly with Mom's local CVS pharmacist to help me understand the likely side effects and possible interactions of medicines more fully.

On at least two occasions during Mom's lengthy dementia journey, I wasn't sure if I should take my mom to the hospital for a medical problem she was experiencing. I called Dr. Ahuja, and because she knew mom so well, she helped me decide whether it was necessary for Mom to go to the hospital. When I thought about taking Mom to the hospital, one of the first questions Dr. Ahuja would ask is "what are your mom's vitals?". If you are taking care of your loved one, the ability to take their vital signs easily and quickly is very important. Taking vitals will give you accurate information about your loved one's condition. It is very easy to do this. The three simple but powerful monitoring devices are:

1. Blood pressure measuring cuff: measures blood pressure; some also report heart rhythms and pulse rate

2. Pulse oximeter ("pulse ox"): measures oxygen level or "oxygen saturation" and pulse

3. Thermometer: measures temperature; I suggest the ear or forehead kind (mouth is too hard or dangerous (biting) to use for most dementia patients. The ear thermometer is a little more accurate than the forehead one. It is not quite as easy but a little more reliable.

There are many different brands and prices for these devices, and they are very easy to use. These three simple tools can be bought at your local pharmacy, medical supply store, or online. You will have peace of mind knowing your loved one's vital signs are acceptable and your loved one is not in immediate danger. The devices can be a critical early warning for you that something more serious needs to be looked at by a doctor. Since your loved one with dementia won't be able to tell you what they are feeling and explain their symptoms to you, these simple vitals measurements will help you know if something is wrong. Taking Mom's blood pressure, oxygen, and temperature helped us on several occasions know that Mom was having a medical problem that needed treatment.

Finding Medical Gurus: When a Good Doctor Is Not Good Enough

Occasionally you or your loved one will have a condition that is very hard to diagnose or treat. A medical condition that is hard to diagnose and treat is especially difficult for a loved one with dementia. A treatable medical condition can linger and cause your loved one ongoing and unnecessary pain, stress, and confusion. Also, going to many doctor visits to find the solution is very hard and alarming for a dementia patient and stressful for you, the care leader.

I learned the hard way that it is very important to find a "medical guru" for hard to diagnose or treat medical conditions. Like all workers, doctors' capabilities fall into a normal bell curve distribution. Having a medical license does not make one physician as good as another. There are poor doctors, average doctors, good doctors, and there are amazingly good doctors (which I call "gurus"). Each medical specialty has a few gurus. It is a good idea for hard to diagnose or to treat conditions to find one of these select "medical gurus." You may be pleasantly surprised that one of these medical gurus practices near where you live.

I learned about the importance of a medical guru when Mom was 70. Before her Alzheimer's symptoms were apparent, Mom had horrible gynecological nerve pain. None of her specialists knew the root cause of her pain and how to treat her. I wish I had found a guru earlier than I did because Mom wouldn't have suffered with pain and the stress of not finding a cure for so long. My mom bravely went to 13 different physicians, all specialists (yes, 13!!!), all over Orange and LA County for this gynecologic condition. We went to gynecologists, urogynecologists, dermatologists, pain specialists, and even a psychiatrist. All these specialists we were told were "good doctors". Finally, after seeing enough of these specialists, a diagnosis emerged: vulvodynia. However, the proposed treatments were all over the map. One even suggested a radical surgery which would have been even more painful than her current pain. We tried a few less drastic treatments, but none of them helped. That was it! I had finally had it, and I knew poor Mom was at her wits end, too. For this condition, good doctors were not good enough.

I decided to do my own research to find the best gynecologist(s) in the world who knew the most about this condition. I frantically searched for specialists who had done research, professional organization presentations, or gotten grants on the topic of vulvodynia. I quickly wrote emails and made calls to hospitals, schools, and research centers all over the country and internationally, too. I discovered that most of the vulvodynia gurus belonged to an organization called The National Vulvodynia Association. I wanted the membership list for this organization to find an expert near me. I contacted the organization, paid my small membership dues, and received the worldwide contact list. I was ready to take Mom anywhere in the world to help relieve the pain she was experiencing. We were blessed because I saw the name of a gynecologist on the Vulvodynia membership list in San Diego, not far from where we lived in Orange County: Dr. Jon Willems, a worldwide expert in vulvodynia and the head of gynecology and obstetrics for Scripps Hospital in San Diego. He conducted seminars and talks on the topic and had research grants for the condition of vulvodynia. Eureka!!! We may have found real help for Mom.

We made an appointment with Dr Willems and drove down to see him for the first time. When I told him that a fellow respected gynecologist suggested that Mom's entire region be removed, I thought he was going to "blow a stethoscope." He was visibly embarrassed, angry, and upset. He said that surgery would not have worked and would have been a horrendous painful disaster. Over many years, I have observed that doctors rarely criticize or question fellow doctors. I have never completely understood why doctors are so afraid of disagreeing with each other. The fact that Dr. Willems was willing to suggest (although he never said it) that this other doctor was the biggest idiot on earth for suggesting that kind of surgery gave me peace of mind that Mom was in good hands. I was ecstatic that we found a truly great doctor who knew exactly how to effectively treat Mom. After trying a series of non-invasive Percutaneous Tibial Nerve Stimulation (PTNS) treatments over only a couple of months, my mom was cured and relieved of all that long term pain. A tiny virtually painless nerve stimulation needle gently placed on her ankle for ten minutes per treatment, believe it or not, cured this horrific stubborn long-term painful gynecological problem. The fact that the other specialists did not know about or did not think of this simple non-invasive solution, which helped Mom so much, still boggles my mind. Dr. Willems demonstrated the power of being compassionately creative; this simple noninvasive nerve treatment worked for another related urologic nerve issue and so he learned that it also worked for Vulvodynia. I was mad at myself that I allowed Mom's pain to go on for so long and had to put her through the horror of going to 13 different "good specialists" when the solution was so simple and painless.

I learned so much from this experience. I can't express to you enough how powerful finding a medical guru is when good doctors can't solve the problem. I don't know if it is the specialist's ego that won't let doctors admit to you or themselves that they don't really know what to do or care enough to take the extra time to find you a medical guru.

I share this medical guru story for two reasons. First, Mom did not have dementia when we went on this wild goose chase for a cure for her gynecological pain. However, once your loved one has dementia, the lack of mobility or their agitation at seeing 13 doctors to solve a condition would be impossible. Sometimes, it can be very difficult to take your dementia loved one to even one. Second, if you suspect something is off about a doctor or you don't find their proposed treatment acceptable (e.g., surgery you don't want your loved one to have), please find a medical guru. It is very likely that the medical guru's treatment idea, because of superior knowledge, experience, and compassionate creativity will be simpler, easier, less invasive, and more effective than the average doctor. It may take a little outside-the-bun research to find someone, but you *can* find these truly gifted doctors. For routine conditions, a good or very good specialist is likely good enough (never accept poor or average doctors on your care team). Believe me, it will be worth the effort to find a medical guru for tough cases. I wish I had learned this earlier for Mom's vulvodynia.

I put this medical guru learning into practice later when Mom did have Alzheimer's and it would be impossible to go to multiple doctors to solve a problem. Mom had developed some lung and breathing issues. Mom's local "good pulmonologist" did a lung scan and prescribed some home nebulizer treatments, antibiotics, and supplemental oxygen. However, the improvements were negligible. He didn't seem to have any other ideas. The red flag went up, and I immediately pressed the "find a medical guru search button." I rapidly identified a top-notch lung guru, not far away, at Cedar Sinai Hospital in Los Angeles. Dr. Chaux was the Director of the Advanced Lung Institute at Cedar Sinai in Los Angeles and had done lung transplants and some of the most advanced lung research in the country. These qualifications, in my mind, set him apart as a "lung guru" for Mom. I was able to schedule an appointment with him surprisingly quickly. It is a paradox that you can't see an average or good specialist for months, but you can see a national leader on lung care or vulvodynia in a matter of a week or two.

On Mom's first visit, Dr. Chaux prescribed a machine that did chest compressions at home. This was a machine that was used for COPD, but he thought it would help with Mom's condition, too. Two tubes would go from the pumping machine into a vest that Mom would wear. It was very easy to put the vest on Mom and secure the tubes so that the machine could then pump air into the vest and shake her chest. The shaking motion loosened all the phlegm in her chest and stimulated her lungs to work better. He told us to use the machine for just 15 minutes each day. Medicare covered this very expensive lung shaker with a prescription from Dr. Chaux. When I ordered the machine from the Medical Device supplier, the salesperson asked us what color we wanted the vest to be and, of course we chose pink (Mom's favorite color). Within 48 hours, the lung shaker machine arrived at the house; I worried that Mom might resist the shaking movement. I was wrong because she loved the shaking. She loved the color of the vest and the shaking motion; the sound of the machine seemed to relax her and give her comfort. Mom even fell asleep during some of the treatments.

Within a week (yes, only a week), Mom's lungs were much better; she had less congestion and breathed more easily. We kept giving Mom these simple short treatments at home throughout the rest of her Alzheimer's journey, and her lungs were clear from that point forward. Like the simple non-invasive PTNS treatments for Mom's vulvodynia, using a chest compressor machine was such a simple non-invasive solution yet was crucial to Mom's health. This again is the power of the medical guru at work. Both medical guru solutions were simple, non-invasive, common sense, and compassionately creative; they ingeniously applied what worked for a related condition to Mom's condition.

Our wonderful caregivers, our good doctors, and a few select medical gurus helped Mom to live longer and happier. Please, accept only the very best doctors you can find; don't ever put up with even average physician help. Also, be sure to find a medical guru when your regular doctor does not quickly diagnose and effectively treat your loved one.

Other Key Medical Specialists on Your Team

Sometimes, you will need a specialist other than a neurologist on your loved one's medical care team. In addition to your PCP and neurologist, there are many other medical specialists from cardiology to urology to oncology, hematology, and others your loved one may need to see. Mom needed a couple of medical specialists on her team to take care of a few of her other medical conditions.

Pulmonologist. Thankfully, we found Dr. Chaux, the lung guru, and she got us the chest compression machine. However, later, despite being very careful with her eating, Mom got a case of aspiration pneumonia for a short time. Your loved one with dementia is likely to need a pulmonologist at some point on their team. Alzheimer's and dementia patients can have problems swallowing their food carefully correctly. If your loved one has a swallowing problem, and there is no one around to assist them with eating and drinking, it is very easy for them to get little pieces of food or liquid drawn into their lungs. Once the food or liquid gets trapped and starts to accumulate in the lungs, your loved one could develop a dangerous case of aspiration pneumonia, resulting in a hospital stay. Dementia patients can also get one of the other types of pneumonia from not moving or not being mobile enough in the later stages of the disease. Because pneumonia can be fatal to your loved one, keeping them moving, eliminating a fall risk, and keeping them away from others who have a contagious illness (especially those who live together in a facility or community) is the key to staying healthy and pneumonia free. Pulmonologists are the lung doctors who will be able to diagnose and treat the different kinds of pneumonias or any other breathing issues your loved one may face.

Urologist. Dementia patients, especially women, can also be prone to urinary tract and related infections (UTI). During part of Mom's journey, she experienced a few repeated UTIs. These infections can be life threatening, highly painful, and cause a tremendous amount of confusion and agitation to a dementia patient. Unfortunately, your loved one will be unsuccessful at telling you if they have symptoms of a UTI.

With a big focus on cleaning, hygiene, and frequent toilet visits, Mom's caregivers reduced and finally eliminated the occurrences of her UTI's. I was immensely grateful that our wonderful caregivers knew both the color and smell of the type of urine that indicated she had a UTI. We quickly knew whether she was safe. With our super caregivers, we were virtually able to eliminate UTIs, a problem, in addition to less than stellar cleaning, that causes elderly dementia patients to develop repeated dangerous UTI's is not being able to tell you that they must urinate. If they are not taken to the bathroom frequently enough, they usually either hold it in or sit in their urine for too long. If either of these issues occur, or improper cleaning, it is very likely that patients will develop a painful and dangerous UTI. Unfortunately, if there aren't enough caregivers in your home or a care facility, and your loved one isn't getting much individual care, UTIs will be the result.

A good urologist for your loved one certainly helps and can hopefully eliminate this problem. If your loved one gets chronic UTI's, first investigate the quality and coverage of their caregivers. Are your loved one's caregivers being highly proactive and timely in cleaning your loved one thoroughly and professionally? Also, a urologist can prescribe a low prophylactic dose of antibiotics for a period to help avoid these infections. Before our super caregivers came and saved the day, Mom's urologist gave her this low prophylactic dose of antibiotics, which helped reduce her UTIs. Also, a supplement that Mom took that helped minimize dangerous UTI's is called D-Mannose.

Other Physicians. Additional medical specialists may be needed based on the medical conditions your loved one has. These may include cardiologists, oncologists, hematologists, or others.

Mom, for example, also needed a cardiologist to occasionally monitor her due to an earlier heart valve issue and some mild blockage of a carotid artery as well as elevated blood pressure. Cardiovascular issues are often connected to vascular dementia. Mom's slightly blocked carotid artery was a likely cause of the vascular dementia part of her Alzheimer's and vascular dementia diagnosis. Mom had a very good cardiologist: Dr. Myla, who was very knowledgeable.

My Respect Hot Button

As you evaluate potential physicians for your loved one, their experience, education, availability, track record, creative compassion, communication skills, phone access and service mindset are all very important considerations as you choose doctors for your loved one's A+ physician team.

One of my selection hot buttons was also how the person treats Mom during an appointment. Your loved one may not be able to communicate to the doctor about their needs and what they are feeling at the time, and you will probably have to answer most or all the doctor's questions about your loved one's symptoms and care. That was my care leader role. However, if a doctor acted like Mom was invisible and only talked about her and made no effort to communicate with her directly or treat her with caring and respect, then they did not pass the "respect test" to be Mom's doctor or any other service provider. I know Mom felt when someone was cold, rude, or acted like she was invisible or less than a person. I could tell, even without speech, that she had hurt feelings. Regardless of her condition, Mom was human, special, sensitive, and compassionate and understood when a person was disrespectful.

Mom's neurologists, Dr. Pierce and Dr. Clarke, like many of Mom's other outstanding regular doctors, were exceptional at making Mom feel appreciated and important. I really valued the doctors who appropriately treated Mom with respect and care and spoke personally with her (even when Mom could not answer as she lost her capacity for speech). They would compliment Mom on her clothing, jewelry, or hair; you could tell Mom was happy when they did that. If I wanted to speak with Mom's neurologist, in detail, about Mom, we would step aside into a private area to talk. This way we were not talking about her in front of her. During these times, a nurse or Mom's caregiver would talk with Mom or play a fun game.

I liked when a doctor would appropriately show respect and care personally for Mom. Mom's spirit, soul, mind, and heart were still there; Mom was still a precious child of God. Your loved one's physicians (and any other care provider) should show respect and speak directly to them even if they cannot communicate well or at all. I suggest you also consider adding this "respect" selection criterion when you choose care providers for your loved one.

Chapter Summary

A strong medical team for your loved one is key not just for longevity but also for happiness. If your loved one is sick or in pain, they will not be very happy. Finding the best medical providers that you can is very important.

1. Your loved one should have a neurologist who is very experienced with dementia and Alzheimer's diseases. This kind of neurologist is one of the most important players on your doctor team. They can guide you and show you with what the normal dementia progression is like for your loved one. They can help you understand how medications and treatments prescribed by other doctors will affect your loved one with dementia. They, along with your primary doctor, can help you assess any potential tradeoffs and side effects of medical treatments or recommend a hospital visit for your loved one with dementia.

2. Your PCP, provided they are highly accessible, is also a key team member. As your loved one's dementia progresses, mobility and going to the doctor will become more difficult. You want to be able to call your PCP especially for their point of view on prescriptions and for the routine medical care your loved one needs. It is important that you can easily talk directly to the doctor on the phone (not just their office staff). This will save your loved one from unnecessarily becoming agitated about having to hurry up and come in for a visit, or worse, wait weeks for an appointment.

3. You may need to find a real medical guru on occasion. As your loved one's dementia progresses, it will be more stressful and difficult to go to the doctor. If your loved one has a condition that is hard to diagnose or treat, don't delay; find a doctor who is a guru in that field. It is costly, stressful, and possibly dangerous for your loved one to have to see multiple doctors to properly diagnose and treat a medical problem. Quickly find someone

who knows what to do. To find a medical guru for your loved start with going online; find doctors who publish, speak, and get grants in the medical area your loved one needs. They are often associated with a university or the top medical centers and are sometimes in urban areas. Don't assume a medical research guru or professor does not see patients. Almost all these medical professors and researchers also see patients.

4. I used to think all doctors were the same; but they are not. Like workers in all other fields, there are poor doctors, average doctors, good doctors, great doctors, and then amazing medical gurus. Find the very best doctors, and they will help your loved one live longer, healthier, and be happier. You will have peace of mind, too.

Making the Most of Doctors' Appointments: The Critical Questions List

Once you feel good about your loved one's team of physicians, how do you make sure the appointments with each are as effective and productive as possible? One problem is that many doctors are rushed. There are many reasons doctors give for why appointments are rushed, including how they schedule their day and weeks and how many patients they want (or need) to fit in. Some doctors work only four days a week, into which they jam all their patients. Also, our medical insurance reimbursement system bears some of the responsibility. Insurance companies are creating a large incentive for doctors to rush through patients. Let me explain why. When my Sicilian grandmother (Nanny) was a seamstress, she said that where she worked had a "piece work" system. Piece work is a type of employment arrangement in the garment industry in which a worker is paid a fixed amount of money for each garment sewn (for example 50 cents or a dollar a shirt). Because of this my grandmother worked fast and on as many garments as possible to make enough money to help take care of her family. The more garment pieces you sewed, the more money you could make. Medical insurance payment methods, in this country, are unfortunately much like this "piece work" garment system. Doctors, like piece workers, are paid largely by the number of patients they see. The more patients they see, the more money they make. Also, the insurance company might pay the doctor $150 for a certain visit condition and earmark that associated visit as a 20-minute appointment (a more complex visit might be $250 for a 40-minute visit). However, if you can see three patients in that same 20-minute window the doctor will receive three insurance payments of $150 instead of just the one $150 visit that the insurance pays for. The insurance company won't know the doctor saw three patients instead of one. You, the patient, become a little like a garment, where the more patients seen in less time, the more money they make. You or the insurance company can't do much about this, or can you?

Regardless of our piecework medical insurance system or any other reason, your important job as care leader is to slow down the doctor to truly help you and your loved one. Slowing down the doctor means that you will be able to communicate more about your loved one's health so they can provide a more thoughtful diagnosis and treatment plan. I have spoken to doctors about this, and many believe they still can provide great care in that shorter amount of time. However, I think many don't know what they don't know (a common problem I have found for executives in corporate America as well as many other overly confident professionals).

Hopefully, you have chosen an empathetic and highly skilled doctor. Once you are in the exam room, you cannot change the baseline competence of that doctor, but you can impact the thoughtfulness and thoroughness of their care. A good way to do this is by having a specific prepared list of questions to bring to each appointment. Here is the list of questions that I found very helpful. I often adjust or combine these questions depending on the situation, but I drew in some way from the essence of this list for every one of Mom's doctor's appointments.

Questions List for Doctor Appointments

1. With these symptoms, what do you think is going on with Mom? What else could it be?

2. What could be causing this? What else might be causing it?

3. Why do you think this is the cause? And why did you rule out other possible causes?

4. As you look over Mom's medication list, could any of these medications or their potential side effects be causing her symptoms?

5. What are the possible treatments for Mom's condition?

6. Which treatment do you recommend? Why is this a better treatment than other possible treatments?

7. What are the potential side effects and risks with this suggested treatment?

8. How might Mom's age or Alzheimer's affect the success or the risks of this treatment?

9. How many of your patients who are Mom's age and have dementia have had this treatment or medicine? What were those patients' experiences with it? Was it successful with all of them or only some of them? What side effects did they experience?

10. How long will it take for this treatment (or medication) to work? And what are the other keys to it being successful?

11. What should we look for as Mom starts this treatment?

12. How and when do we follow up with you on her treatment (or medication)?

You can probably see how the thoroughness and the time these questions take might annoy less creative and compassionate doctors. They must slow down and think or maybe even do some research to answer them. Should you care if your doctor is a little annoyed by these questions? I encourage you to say no to yourself about that. If your doctor does not regularly know or think about these questions or does not have the courtesy to tell you their thoughts about these questions (assuming they have them), then it is time to look for a better doctor. You as care leader have more important things to worry about (like your loved one's care and your peace of mind) than worry about a very highly paid professional being annoyed by the thoroughness of your questions.

As you can see from the essence of some of these questions, treatments and medications often work differently and have different impacts on older patients and dementia patients than younger patients. There are numerous examples of the different impacts that various treatments and medications have on dementia patients. One common example of one of these is anesthesia. Anesthesia has very little negative impact on young people or even very healthy older people but can be dangerous for elderly loved ones with dementia. A dementia patient has very limited cognitive reserve capacity, and anesthesia often saps the limited cognitive reserve. Anesthesia can often be a negative influence on your loved one's already diminished mental capability. Narcotic sleeping pills, pain pills, tranquilizers, and many decongestants have the same negative impact on your loved one's cognitive brain function. The commercials on television, after listing the numerous risks and side effect of many pills and procedures, often say, "Your doctor has likely prescribed this because the benefits outweigh the risks." This may be true for younger people, but the risk calculus differs for elderly dementia patients. Make sure your doctor has plenty of experience with older patients and specifically older patients with dementia. They need to know whether the benefits of a certain medicine or treatment really outweigh the risks for your specific and unique loved one with dementia.

If I had a hunch the doctor did not have a lot of experience with this medication or treatment for elderly dementia patients, I would ask Mom's seasoned neurologists if they thought this suggested treatment or medication would be safe for Mom with her Alzheimer's. This would often shed important light on the potential negative impact for Mom specifically.

Remember, doctors hate to criticize recommendations by other doctors, so if one physician prescribes something, another doctor may be reluctant to say that medicine is not a good idea for your loved one. To prompt greater honesty, I sometimes framed the question like this: "I am thinking about giving [medication name or treatment] to Mom." I found asking the question hypothetically, not surprisingly, yielded more openness & honesty from doctors than if you say another doctor, especially if they know the other doctor, is suggesting the medicine or treatment. Please don't underestimate doctors' fear of disagreeing with each other. I know playing these kinds of physician games seem silly, but it is very important to know what doctors *honestly* think about a treatment or medicine recommended for your loved one. Care more about what is likely to happen given your loved one's age, health, and specific medical conditions, including dementia.

Having such a list of questions for your doctor is key to encouraging you and the doctor to slow down and be as thoughtful and caring as possible about your special loved one. If your doctor is a real speedster and you don't seem to be able to get through your list of questions or have a hard time seeing yourself asking some of these questions because of the doctor's perceived busyness, I have two tips to slow down any physician sprinters and help you get answers to these questions. First, print out copies of your list of questions; then, actually hand one copy to the doctor and keep one for yourself. Tell the doctor at the outset these are your questions you would like addressed in today's visit. Ask the doctor to look over the list. I found this works well for the speedsters who wouldn't let me finish my questions by just asking them verbally. Handing your physician the written list will also help if you feel a little awkward (which, I hope, with time you will learn not to be) asking any of them verbally. Occasionally, a doctor's need for speed would fluster me, so handing the list to the doctor helped make sure I didn't forget an important question. Even when I handed the doctor the list, a true gold medal sprinter physician would skip questions either to get out faster, consider the questions unimportant, or just not feel like answering them. Even with a handout, you may still have to blurt out, "What do you think about question #4, Doctor?" Handing them a copy of the written list enables you to do that.

My second tip is even bolder. I have only had to do this once, when the doctor was a true gold medal contender for the "50-yard get out of the exam room dash." If you hand the doctor the list of questions and he/she still does not answer them and looks like he is ready to rush out the door, simply stand in the doorway. Because your loved one is likely to be sitting on the exam table, I would quietly slide over and stand in the doorway after the doctor came in. I am not suggesting you play NFL blocker and physically block the doctor from leaving the room (although that might be interesting). However, I found that the visual cue of you standing in the doorway and potentially blocking the exit path helped the physician think twice about sprinting out the door. I know it is a little bizarre to have to block a doorway, but you have the right to and should get the best care possible for your loved one. You and your loved one deserve the respect of getting every question you have answered thoroughly and to make sure the doctor is really thinking through care for your loved one.

We all know doctors are important and do deserve a lot of respect, but remember they are just human like you and me. Have respect for your doctor, but do not let them get away with the bad behavior, acting too busy, being a bully, or being arrogant. If you have any doubt that your physician is very human, let me remind you that a University of Chicago study (2017) found that almost 50% of people in the United States have been either directly harmed by a medical mistake or know someone close to them that was harmed by a medical mistake. See, physicians are very human. To let your doctor get away with any of these bad behaviors can be dangerous for your loved one. You need to make sure the doctor takes all the time necessary for a thorough and caring visit that includes all your questions and includes respect for your loved one and for you. too. You are your loved one's champion, and if doctors do not give both of you adequate respect, you have to make sure they do.

Paradoxically, I have found the medical gurus took significantly more time examining Mom and answering my questions. The medical gurus were, from my experience, more respectful, empathetic, and humble than even "good" doctors. The gurus took more time with Mom perhaps because they were just more caring, empathetic, creative, and wanted to be "of true service" to their patients. This extra compassion and creativity probably is what made these medical gurus the best doctors in their field. When you care more, you become more creative, competent, and more compassionate. If you have a 50-yard dasher, consider finding a doctor who is a champion doctor, not a champion speedster. Again, I hope you pick the best and not settle for average healthcare for your loved one. The very best physicians are worth finding. Please remember, you and your loved one deserve the very best. The very best will help you achieve breakthrough care and help your loved one live happier, healthier and longer.

Chapter Summary

Physicians are a very important part of your caregiving team and are crucial to the Breakthrough Care System. There is a strong link between physical health and cognitive health. When a body is healthy, the mind is much more likely to be healthy. Your loved one will be happier when they feel better. Diabetes, heart disease, high blood pressure, excessive weight, sleep apnea, poor nutrition, and other medical problems are all linked to dementia. Staying out of the hospital is important, but some surgeries may be necessary for your loved one. However, surgeries, anesthesia, and long hospital stays pose alarming risks and problems for the elderly and especially dementia patients. Mistakes and problems in the hospital are a lot more common than most people think. Make sure surgery is truly necessary because they can be dangerous. Find a medical guru to confirm that surgery is necessary; there may be state-of-the-art solutions that are not surgical. Even routine surgery is risky for an elderly dementia patient. It is much better for dementia patients to be medically healthy and stay out of the hospital. Your doctors, if they are exceptional, can help your loved one stay healthy, stay out of the hospital, and maintain a positive connection between body and mind. This is my wish for you and your loved one.

1. An important care leader role is to make sure you find the best doctors for your team and make sure they slow down and really focus thoroughly and thoughtfully on your loved one's care. Like your direct caregivers, your loved one's doctors need to show

compassion, creativity, skill, and keen ability to observe and really tune into your loved one's symptoms and needs.

2. Some doctors are very rushed in their care. To help them slow down and really focus on your loved one, a good list of physician questions, like the one in this chapter, can help you and the doctor. Often, handing the doctor a copy of your written list of questions works best to slow them down and might be easier for you.

3. If you are frequently frustrated because your doctor is not very accessible for appointments or phone calls, you always feel rushed by the doctor, or you often leave without your questions answered, it is time to find a better doctor for your loved one. There are excellent doctors out there who are highly accessible, more empathetic, and creative and who will take the time you want and need.

4. Doctors are essential to breakthrough care. Don't settle for an average physician for your loved one's team. Find an excellent doctor and even a medical guru. You and your loved one need and deserve that for breakthrough care results. Doctors are humans just like you! You are an empowered care leader and your loved one needs the best doctors to live longer and be happier. Some doctors are hard to lead, but I know your empowered care leadership will ensure your physician team members provide your loved one incredible care.

CHAPTER 22

Leading Non-Physician Specialists on Your Team

Some family members will start out caring for their loved one at home and then place them in a facility when things get hard. Others may keep their loved one in a facility almost or all their entire journey. If you want to keep your loved one at home for some or all their dementia journey, please remember this: **any** *kind of medical service, supply, equipment, or therapy that you can get in a rehab or other facility, you can also get at home!* I emphasize this because few people know this. I did not know this with my grandmother years ago; I assumed my grandmother needed to be in a rehab facility after her hospital visit to have physical and other therapies. I was wrong. Here is another paradox, I found with my mom, the opposite was true. I found even better and more available medical and related therapies, services, and supplies at home than those in a facility. Mom used these important services and therapies regularly at home over her entire long Alzheimer's journey. These therapies really helped Mom live longer, healthier, and happier at home. I received the names of amazing and talented "mobile at home" specialists from our home care agencies, from the Alzheimer's Association, and even from the hospital.

I wish I had known this secret about there being so many home therapies and services when my grandmother was needing them. I would have kept my grandmother at home, too. If I had known that, I believe my grandmother might have lived longer and happier. I believe some of our loved ones, if they had all the necessary help, services, and therapies would consistently rather be at home than a rehab, nursing home, or related facility. It is a shame that more people don't know you can get all this good help at home; this makes caring for your loved one at home much more doable than most people think. The extra bonus is that insurances like Medicare will pay for all these home medical specialists just like they would in a rehab facility or nursing home. Now, you know this secret, too. Please don't keep it a secret; tell everyone you know so they can benefit from this as well.

Here are a few of the therapies and services Mom took advantage of at home. The best way to find these incredible mobile specialists is through referrals from home care agencies or your local Alzheimer's associations or hospitals. They usually know the most terrific people who do at home therapies or other at home services. All these therapies and services will really help your loved one whether they are at home or in a facility.

Mobile Physical Therapist

Having a physical therapist on an ongoing basis for Mom was crucial because the mind and body connection was an important part of her journey. Alzheimer's and other dementias affect your loved one's ability to walk and complete other physical activities. The longer you help your loved one stay mobile, the healthier and happier they will be. Mom's physical therapy helped her with walking and balance and made it easier for her to go on fun outings every day. Mobility likely helped Mom live longer and gave her a happier outlook. Weekly physical therapy, especially for the last half of her journey was key to her success in these two areas. Mobility also helped with Mom's lung function and decreased the likelihood of her getting pneumonia or other ailments that stem directly from inactivity. Usually, facilities only prescribe physical therapy if there is an injury. An experienced home therapist knows how to work with your insurance company to optimize the need for ongoing physical therapy for dementia patients due to decreased mobility. This will then help keep your loved mobile and active. Because of the significant walking and balance issues associated with Alzheimer's disease, ongoing weekly preventative physical therapy helps avoid a fall that would paradoxically *then require* physical therapy.

We found an amazing home physical therapist who was recommended to us by Mom's orthopedic doctor. His name was Christian. He came to the house weekly for ten weeks at a time a couple of times a year during the first half of my mom's Alzheimer's journey. He then came every week, like clockwork, for the second half of Mom's long Alzheimer's journey. Helping Mom weekly for years was the reason Mom, unlike many other dementia patients, was able to walk throughout her entire Alzheimer's journey. Christian would work on strengthening Mom's legs and arms, stretching her limbs and hips, and working on her balance. In addition to being highly capable he was always patient with Mom's Alzheimer's. He knew how to make the therapy fun. He would sing and play music for Mom while he worked on Mom. This fun approach to therapy really helped Mom look forward to physical therapy every week and she smiled from ear to ear when they worked together.

Yes, your loved one can go to a physical therapy center to do therapy, but as Alzheimer's gradually advances, getting your loved one to a center may get more difficult. Due to this increasing difficulty of getting out, you and your loved might be tempted to give up on doing physical therapy. With a home therapist this won't happen, and your loved one may also get much more 1:1 attention than in a center. Medicare and other insurances will pay for physical therapy at home.

Mobile Dentist

There are studies that show that good dental hygiene can reduce dementia risks. Dental procedures can be tough on your loved one with dementia. Keeping your mouth open for a long time can be very hard for anyone but is particularly hard for dementia patients. Somewhere in the middle of Mom's Alzheimer's journey, she developed a wanting-to-bite issue, where she would occasionally bite down on utensils, thermometers, and dentists. I recall a visit to our family dentist who had a difficult time cleaning her teeth because Mom bit down on the instruments.

I realized I had to do something to help keep Mom's teeth and gums healthy. I called a couple of our wonderful home care agencies, and one agency knew a dentist who would come to your home or facility. I then called this at-home dentist and asked her to see Mom. Kim, who owned Smiles on the Run Dentistry, arrived. I noticed she had all the equipment and supplies, just like any dental office would have. I helped her bring her equipment into the house, and she was wonderful with Mom. We happened to have a lazy boy chair that went back just like the chair in a dental office; it worked great. Not only was Kim an empathetic and capable dentist, but Mom really felt very calm with her. She was very patient with Mom, and she knew the idiosyncrasies of dementia patients' behavior. I know it seems impossible to make dental work fun, but Kim did exactly that. I could tell Mom liked Kim and therefore did what Kim wanted her to do. Because of Kim's wonderful skills, knowledge of dementia, and loving attitude, Mom, thankfully, did not bite down on her instruments or on Kim's fingers. Between Kim's attitude and skills and the comfort of being at home, the dental appointments went beautifully, with no problems. Again, Mom's dental insurance paid for Kim.

Dementia patients often can't tell you when something is wrong with their teeth or gums. A doctor will tell you that dental problems and medical health problems are closely connected. Also, if your loved one has mouth pain it will negatively affect their happiness and likely their longevity. Healthy and clean teeth and gums can prevent further medical problems and lessen behavioral issues like agitation, aggression, or aggravation caused by mouth pain. Once again, cognitive, physical, and emotional health are closely linked. I have heard of people, unfortunately, putting their dementia loved one under anesthesia to keep them calm just for a routine dental procedure like regular cleanings or a minor cavity. Anesthesia is usually very bad for dementia patients, and administering it unnecessarily can accelerate cognitive decline. It would be much better to find an excellent home care dentist like Kim, someone with lots of empathy, creativity, and dementia care experience, full of love, care, skills, and fun. This is much better than knocking your loved one out. Like our wonderful home physical therapist, Kim was a key member of Mom's Breakthrough Care Team

Mobile Podiatrist

A home podiatrist was another important specialist for Team Mom. As you may know, your toenails get harder to cut as you age. Bad toenails or other foot issues can limit the mobility of your loved one. We know that continued walking and exercise are key for physical, cognitive, and emotional health. At one point in Mom's journey, Marina and I realized that neither we, nor our caregivers, could effectively cut Mom's toenails and provide foot care for her callouses, corns and her overall foot health. We decided to call on our home agencies again. One gave us the name of an excellent mobile podiatrist, Dr. Stockard. We called, and he came to our house and gently, thoroughly, and patiently cared for Mom's feet. He also knew how to keep Mom from squirming while he worked on her feet. Once every two months, throughout Mom's entire Alzheimer's journey, he came to the house to check on and care for Mom's feet. Dr. Stockard was an important part of keeping mom physically active, healthy, happy, and comfortable. Dr. Stockard's home visits were covered by Mom's Medicare and Medicare supplement insurances. Some people have told me that some Medicare Advantage Plans may not cover some of these home medical therapies. If that is the case, you may want to consider getting your loved one the core Medicare coverage and add a Medicare supplement to get everything covered no matter where your loved one is. This is an important consideration in choosing your loved one's medical insurance. If you are taking care of your loved one at home or even in a facility, these extra special mobile medical therapies and services are critical to achieving breakthrough results.

Mobile Hair Stylist

Hair cutting is another service you can get at home. One of our agencies gave us the name of a lovely person to cut and style Mom's hair. It was quite easy and comfortable for Mom to get her hair cut at home. Mom tended to squirm and wiggle in the chair when she was getting a haircut. The first hairstylist whom we tried couldn't handle Mom's movements. She became visibly frustrated and upset. We let her go because she was not compassionate, creative, or tuned into Mom enough to be effective. She did not have much experience or patience with Alzheimer's patients. Alzheimer's and dementia patients commonly squirm if they must sit for a while. You don't want your squirming loved one to get a scissor wound due to an inexperienced or frustrated hair stylist. Mom's new home stylist had a lot of clients with dementia. Instead of becoming frustrated with Mom's squirming, her experience and creative empathy allowed her magically to move fluidly with Mom's moving while cutting her hair. I noticed how safely (it was like magic) she cut Mom's hair even while Mom was moving around in the chair. She did not scold Mom; she moved with Mom gracefully to cut her hair.

Mom was very happy, self-satisfied, and cute after she got her haircut. She would look at herself in her bathroom mirror and give herself a big smile. Our wonderful caregivers would tell her how beautiful she was, and it was heartwarming to see Mom smile and be so happy, loving how she looked. It was like the way Mom would admire her special outfits in the mirror when our wonderful caregivers dressed her in a cute dress or skirt. Mom's smile would light up the room and make everyone else smile, too. Even though Mom couldn't speak, you could really see her glow with delight. Mom's home stylist did a great job keeping Mom looking beautiful and her feeling happy. With the right person, it is easy and safe for your loved one to get a haircut at home. Mom's home stylist was another important member of Team Mom.

Other Important At-Home Mobile Services

Services that Mom had at home very late in her journey were home respiratory care, home blood draw, home swallowing therapy, home nursing, and a general practitioner. These incredible mobile specialists all came to our home, and in addition to being technically excellent, they really knew the unique challenges of creatively and compassionately caring for a dementia patient. Medicare paid for all these home medical services and any medical equipment needed, all in the comfort and safety of our home.

If your loved one is in a facility, you can also get all these travelling medical and other services to come to your loved one's facility. If the facility does not provide you with each of these mobile specialists, with your care leader superpower search skills, you can find wonderful mobile experts through a home care agency, hospital, or Alzheimer's organization. It is always good to do a little of your own sourcing because even if a facility has some of these services, it is good to be ready with a backup in case someone the facility provides either does not meet your high standards of care or won't come as frequently as you want to proactively prevent problems (like physical therapy). A good facility will allow you to bring in your own mobile specialists or your own private caregivers.

Finding mobile professionals who know dementia and are motivated to engage your loved one in a caring, creative, and positive way really enhances your loved one's physical, cognitive, and emotional health. With relative ease, I found all these wonderful people to come to the house. They individually and collectively made a huge positive difference for Mom. I was blessed and grateful for all our brilliant at-home mobile specialists.

Chapter Summary

1. There are many important mobile and at-home services that your loved one will benefit from over their dementia journey. These include a physical therapist, a podiatrist, a dentist, a hair stylist, and others. Please remember, every kind of service, therapist, piece of equipment, or medical specialist that is available in any facility is also available in the comfort of your home.

2. Finding these excellent mobile specialists with extensive dementia experience ensures that your loved one not only gets the direct benefit of the help but also gets the additional benefit of focused 1:1 treatment. With exclusive at-home services, versus a center, the mobile specialist will get to know and observe the special needs of your loved one well through one-on-one treatment. At home, they will come to know your loved one better and therefore are more likely to be able to provide the "magic" part

of outstanding care, treating your loved one with patience, creativity, positive energy, comfort, stimulation, and fun. Look for people who can do the latter part, too (they are out there). The first place to look for first-rate mobile specialists is through a home care agency. Working with more than one agency, as with caregivers, will give you access to even more and better mobile specialists. Alzheimer's Associations and hospitals are also good sources to find wonderful mobile specialists.

3. Getting these services at home where things are comfortable and more familiar will also lead to your loved one being less agitated, more comfortable, and less exposed to viruses and germs. This, in turn, will make the service more effective, safe, and enjoyable.

4. Most insurances, including core Medicare, will pay for all the medical therapeutic-related home services.

Breakthrough Pillar #4

Powerful Brain

Nutrition & Medication

A good brain healthy diet, vitamins, and supplements, as well as key medications for brain and body played an important part in Mom's living longer and happier. Most experts agree that a good brain-and-body healthy diet contributes to overall cognitive and physical health. Unfortunately, for a variety of reasons, you may not be able to get your loved one all the powerful nutrients needed through diet only. This was true for my mom. Fortunately, for most of the nutritional pillars that I could not give Mom through her diet, reputable nutritional supplements filled the gaps.

The medical community is not 100% aligned on the positive impact of some supplements for brain health. However, there is some evidence behind all the supplements I gave Mom; the good news is that I observed that these supplements collectively helped Mom a great deal. Do I know exactly what aspects of Mom's nutritional program led precisely to individual aspects of her cognitive and physical longevity and happiness? No, I do not, but that didn't matter to me because I saw Mom benefitting from them. Recall my mission was giving Mom a longer, healthier, and happier life, and Mom's nutrition seemed to be contributing to that. Nutrition, supplements, and medications are important, but they are only one part of the Breakthrough Care System. Many small components coming together made a big positive impact.

Best Brain and Body Enhancing Food and Nutrition

Experts agree the Mediterranean Diet, the MIND diet, and similar diets are good for cognitive and physical health. The essence of these diets is to eat more fruits, vegetables, whole grains, legumes, nuts, seafood, herbs, and olive oil. These diets all tell us to eat less poultry, eggs, and cheese. These diets also recommend that we should only very rarely or not at all eat red meat, sugar and sugar sweetened beverages, refined grains, refined oils and fats, and other processed foods. This type of diet not only helps brain function but also heart health, it reduces cancer risk and helps to regulate blood pressure and blood sugar. These diets are a huge win. The body, brain, and emotions are connected systems and therefore it should be no surprise that what is good for the heart is good for the brain and good for our overall emotional wellness and happiness. Dr. Sanjay Gupta in his excellent book, *Keep Sharp,* discusses the science behind why our diet is so important to reducing dementia risk. In the book, he references studies by Dr. Richard Isaacson, who runs a reputable dementia prevention clinic. Dr. Isaacson found that patients who have dementia already can reduce the severity of symptoms through diet and other lifestyle changes.

Just like for Mom and many other dementia patients, it is common to lose some ability to effectively chew, swallow, and digest most meats, even if they are chopped up in small pieces. Mom benefited greatly by eliminating red meat in her diet. By eliminating red meat altogether, we reduced her choking risk, and simultaneously added better cognitive and physical health. Because Mom eliminated red meat completely, it was important for her to have enough protein from other sources. I started giving Mom whey-based protein in her soups, shakes, and oatmeal. I learned that whey-based forms of protein supplements gave Mom uncomfortable gas and bloating. I switched to a plant-based protein supplement which worked much better. For even more protein in her diet, I added healthy organic lentil soup as a base food and added the plant-based protein powder. Lentil soup has protein, fiber, minerals, and vitamins. I decided to make a big pot of lentil soup every few days. It is thick but not too thick and is therefore not only nutritious but also a great meal for your loved one with dementia who might have difficulty swallowing other types of food. For patients who have a hard time swallowing, "thick" liquids are often prescribed by various doctors and nutritionists because "thin" liquids are too difficult for dementia patients who are losing their swallowing coordination and could easily aspirate thinner liquids into their lungs. Blended lentil soup offers a wonderful consistency, and my mom swallowed and digested the different kinds of lentil soups very well. Lentil soup was also a good base for me to blend in or add other healthy ingredients like broccoli, sweet potatoes, psyllium husk powder (fiber), and other brain and body healthy vegetables and supplements. The lentil soup base made these other nutritious ingredients soft enough for Mom to eat safely.

Oatmeal in the morning was also good for similar reasons. It was healthy and a good consistency for swallowing, plus I could add blueberries or other healthy brain-and-body supplements for Mom. Other nutritious foods Mom liked that were safe to swallow were cut-up pears and bananas in the morning. For lunch, I added the inside of a soft cooked sweet potato, riced cauliflower, peas, and plant protein powder to a bowl of lentil soup. Occasionally, I would prepare very finely diced, marinated, and cooked chicken pieces softened with low sodium broth. If I thought the soft chicken was still too hard to swallow, I would shred it or blend it into the lentil or pea soup.

We added brighter colored fruits and vegetables for Mom's meals because they are filled with more vitamins and nutrition and are better for brain health. Experts say fruits and vegetables with a lot of color have more of the powerful nutrients we need. Mom always had meals with explosions of color, variety, and great taste. Having Mom eat healthy meals and safely enjoy them, with the help of our incredible caregivers, was immensely important to me. The only time we deviated from this ultra-healthy diet was when we went out on our daily adventure and stopped at Sprinkles Ice Cream for a children's scoop of ice cream.. It was a fun outing that Mom eagerly looked forward to every day; it seemed worth the slight deviation from her regular highly nutritious and healthy eating.

Experts agree that getting brain healthy nutrients, vitamins, and minerals from natural food sources is better than getting them from supplements because the body absorbs these nutrients from food more efficiently than in pill form. This made perfect sense to me, and armed with this information, I focused intently on providing Mom with a delicious and terrific natural foods diet.

For patients with dementia, swallowing and chewing can be a challenge, and eating certain brain-healthy foods like nuts and fish can be risky. To make sure Mom did not miss out on any of these important brain-and-body nutrients, I turned to the most reputable brands and the most absorbable forms of supplements.

Nutritional Supplements: Filling the Gaps

Supplements[2] are not regulated so it is important that I found the most reputable suppliers. I also focused on the form of supplements that were the best absorbed by the body and the easiest for Mom to swallow. It seems like powders and liquids can be absorbed better and were also much safer for Mom to swallow than some of the big "horse pills" that are out there. Also, powders and liquid supplements are the most easily added into healthy food bases like soups, smoothies, and oatmeal. I had to crush a couple of vitamin tablets for Mom, but for the most part I was able to find all the desired supplements and vitamins in liquid or powder form.

I researched the following supplements; all had at least some evidence of having brain or body benefit. Mom had lots of great nutrition in her diet, but each of the following supplements filled at least a partial gap in Mom's diet due to her safe swallowing challenges. I encourage you to research each of these nutritional pillars to find out more about how they contribute to brain and body health.

Healthy Brain and Body Vitamins and Supplements

1. Coffee and Green Tea

2. Vitamins: B12, B-Complex, D, E, and a Multi-Vitamin

3. Dark Chocolate Cacao Powder (find brands with the lowest cadmium/other potentially harmful metals)

4. Fish Oil

5. Pre-Biotics and Probiotics

6. Lions Mane

7. Lecithin

8. Selenium

9. MCT Oil

10. CoQ10

---

2. Please note that the rigor by which supplements are tested is not the same as FDA approved prescriptions. You should always talk to your physician(s) before adding supplements and changing your loved one's medications.

11. Acetyl - L-Carnitine

12. Turmeric

13. Alpha gpc choline

Mom had some cardiac and blood pressure issues, and many of these supplements, in addition to helping her cognitively, also had cardiovascular system benefits. Each supplement's separate benefit for Mom may have been very small, but cumulatively they were very important for her.

For many nutritional supplements, like medicines, starting with a very low dose, allowing the body to get used to it, reduces negative reactions and side effects. Because I was also very cautious about interactions among supplements and medicines and each of their potential side effects alone, I would not add a supplement until I was sure there were no negative interactions or side effects. Our body is amazing because it naturally adjusts to many things, so it may just take a little time with a smaller than recommended dose for the body to adjust to taking a certain medicine or supplement. Starting with a very low dose may have helped Mom tolerate these powerful nutrients better; she had no side effects to any of these and was able to receive the benefits from all of them.

I always checked with Mom's neurologists and PCP to be sure both were comfortable with Mom using each vitamin and supplement. I suggest you, too, check with your loved one's doctor before you go forward with a nutrition program like Mom's. I also made sure Mom had very frequent blood tests and would regularly take her vitals to make sure everything together was normal and healthy for Mom.

As you know Alzheimer's disease is a slow death sentence with no known cure. My mindset was that if a supplement or vitamin had "some evidence of benefit" for Mom, and if there were no ill side effects or negative interactions, then it made perfect sense to have her take it on the decent chance it would contribute to her overall cognitive and physical health, longevity, and happiness.

Finally, we know that healthy hydration is important for everyone, especially for elderly patients. Water is important for brain health and for body health. Water transports nutrients and waste products into and out of cells. It is also key for absorption of foods and water-soluble vitamins and supplements. Hydration is important for digestion, excretion, and other important bodily functions. Water also reduces risk for UTIs. I tried to make sure Mom was always drinking enough water. If your loved one resists drinking water, make drinking water a type of game or some kind of fun. Parents of young children know how to do this. Parents make counting sips or bites a game or pretend a bite is an airplane flying into the hangar. Fun games can work for many dementia patients who sometimes become childlike again. Making something fun is a great way to help our loved ones' drink and eat what is important for them and enjoy themselves at the same time. Introducing a fun game can help overall mood, cognition, and create a positive healthy and happy outlook. Hydrating means more urination, which also means taking your loved one to the bathroom more or changing their adult diapers more often. However, please know this extra going to the bathroom work is a good kind of work, helping your loved one's health immensely. Whether at home or in a facility, if caregivers avoid giving your loved one lots to drink because of the work involved with your loved one urinating more, it is time to consider a new caregiver or a new facility. The more trips to the bathroom from drinking more, the healthier your loved one will be. Please don't put up with lazy caregivers.

Mom's good nutrition was a very important part of her overall health and one of the important things that led to extending her life and happiness during her long Alzheimer's journey. As Mom's care leader, I was more than happy to prepare these healthy meals and supplements. Our wonderful caregivers then could focus on being sure Mom ate safely and safely took all her pills, vitamins, and supplements. It was a creative joy for me to experiment as Mom's healthy nutrition chef. Together with my highly talented, fun-loving caregivers we were able to turn Mom's nutrition program into a strong breakthrough care pillar. Because fun was so important to Mom's happiness, her caregivers also made mealtime fun and celebratory. When Mom was having fun and was happy, she was calmer and more willing to eat well and follow her caregivers' guidance for safety. You can see how the breakthrough care components work as a care system, reinforcing each other. For example, fun makes nutritious eating easier and safer, and great nutrition creates physical and emotional well-being, which allows for more fun, energy, mobility, and happiness.

If your loved one is in a facility, you may need to be sure your loved one consistently gets all the wonderful brain-and-body-healthy foods and supplements. I am sure there are facilities that will implement the exact nutrition and supplements program that you want for your loved one. Willingness to implement your desired nutrition program, then, is another important search criterion for you as care leader as you source and evaluate facilities for your loved one.

Your wonderful loved one needs and deserves a special tailored nutrition program to help extend their life and happiness. In the resource section of this book, I list resources where you can find more great information on nutrition, supplements, and other aspects of your loved one's nutrition health. These resources will tell you in detail the type of cognitive benefits and the recommended dosages and possible side effects.

Medications For Dementia and Connected Medical Issues

In addition to diet and brain-enhancing nutritional supplements, Mom's prescriptions were also important. Brain, body, and emotion (calm and happiness) are connected systems. Here are some of Mom's medical challenges related to her Alzheimer's and what prescription medications were prescribed by Team Mom physicians. I share these because they are common for many elderly dementia patients and because brain and body health are often two sides of the same coin.

Dementia Medications

Mom's neurologist suggested that she start *Aricept,* and then soon after she prescribed *Namenda.* These medications represent the two classes of dementia medications that were on the market at the time of Mom's Alzheimer's diagnosis. They are still prescribed to slow the progression of dementia. I started Mom on a below-minimum dose of each and slowly titrated up the dosage to what Mom's neurologist recommended. This approach helped Mom tolerate them beautifully. I believe because we started with the lower doses and very slowly worked up, Mom did not have any of the often-reported side effects that some patients have from these medications.

Today, other medications that show the promise of slowing certain dementias are coming on the market. Your loved one's neurologist can help you decide if any of these new medications might make sense for your loved one. The brain and the brain body connections are extremely complex, and it is wonderful that science is finally beginning to identify more medicines to help with the diseases of Dementia and Alzheimer's. Sadly, there is still no cure, but we are getting a little closer. For now, this Breakthrough Care System, executing many smaller, simultaneous improvements, powerful diet, supplements, medications, physical movement and activity, cognitive stimulation, positivity, familiarity, physical health, fun, and love are the best we have for a longer and happier dementia journey.

Blood Pressure and Heart Concerns

Doctors have discovered that cardiovascular and brain health are closely connected. Unfortunately, Mom had both high blood pressure and some cardiac issues. It was important that they be treated and carefully monitored. *Pravastatin (cholesterol), Atenolol (blood pressure)* and *Tekturna (blood pressure)* were what the cardiologist Dr. Myla prescribed for Mom. Mom also had periodic echo cardiograms to keep an eye on her narrow ceratoid artery. As our loved ones get older, it is not uncommon that cardiac issues arise. It is very important that these be managed by a creatively compassionate and caring cardiologist on your team. This will help heart health, brain health, and longevity.

Anxiety and Agitation

Alzheimer's patients often experience agitation and anxiety during their journey. Mom's agitation and anxiety was milder than most. Marina and I did many things to keep Mom happy and to reduce her anxiety.

Being surrounded with fun, warm, and loving caregivers and family and experiencing a comfortable familiarity living at home with us, I believe, contributed to Mom's minimal agitation and feel-good attitude. Being a little less agitated has so many benefits. It made going out for our daily fun adventure easier and more fun, which lowered agitation and anxiety (another example of the system reinforcing itself). It also made needed doctor visits and important home therapies easier and therefore more frequent, all of which in turn contributed to Mom's overall health and happiness.

I knew that if I could virtually eliminate Mom's agitation and anxiety, Mom would be even happier and healthier. I consulted Mom's neurologists. Because higher doses of many anti-anxiety medications would make Mom's cognitive decline worse, Mom's neurologist suggested that a low dose of the SSRI *Celexa,* an anti-anxiety and antidepressant medication, might have the least negative impact on cognitive reserve of Alzheimer's patients but still would likely take away the small amount of agitation Mom had. I did not want to sedate Mom and was told it wouldn't. We decided to start Mom on the lowest dose of Celexa 10 mg. I cut the pill in half and gave her half of the minimum recommended dose, i.e. 5 mg. The super small dose, together with all of Mom's positive environmental support and fun, reduced her anxiety and agitation to virtually zero and gave her a more consistently calm, positive, and active outlook. Throughout her entire Alzheimer's journey I never had to raise the 5mg. dose of Celexa—the best news of all.

I urge you to be very careful in how you manage your loved one's anxiety and agitation. There is a lot written about nursing homes and other facilities administer sedatives to more than 70% of agitated patients. They tend to administer many strong psychotropic drugs to sedate and calm patients who may just be plain frightened because they are living in an unfamiliar place. Recent articles have called many of these medications "chemical straitjackets" to control patients. Simply spending more 1:1 time creatively and compassionately having fun and being lovingly empathetic would likely work much better. Unfortunately, some of these facilities don't have staffing levels or skills to comfort and keep your loved one happy and calm. It is sad and such a shame that so many patients rapidly decline cognitively and physically from these anti-anxiety drugs due to a lack of appropriate caregivers. If you can create an environment that assists in anxiety reduction and positively stimulates your loved one, there will be no need for these "straight jacket" drugs that cause such a dramatic mental and physical decline.

I did not want any part of a "chemical straight jacket" or sedation for my mom, so the approach of giving her the very slightest boost in her mood with this 5 mg dose of Celexa really seemed to work. I wanted to thread the needle and get near zero agitation for Mom with zero sedating effect. I wanted her natural vibrant, loving light to shine and not be hidden away with by sedation. Thankfully, with my grandmother's help, our former seamstress in heaven, we threaded that needle.

Nighttime Sleeping

Problems sleeping at night are very common with Alzheimer's patients. Alzheimer's patients usually have what is called Sundowner Syndrome, where they stay up at night and then nap in the daytime. Mom would be up at night but did not nap much during the day, either. Lack of sleep is not good for the body or the brain. Mom needed to get more than just occasional sleep, so I tried her on melatonin. This worked to give Mom a little sleep during the night. However, later in Mom's journey, melatonin stopped working well. I contacted Mom's neurologist to find out what else would help her sleep. She suggested Gabapentin for Mom. Because dizziness is a side effect, I started Mom on much less than a minimum dose. A low dose of melatonin with an ultra-low dose of gabapentin worked well together to improve Mom's sleep a little, even late into her Alzheimer's journey. Most important, it did not change Mom's happy personality by over-sedating her.

You might ask what about Ambien or other prescription sleeping pills that have a narcotic effect. The big problem with these classes of sleeping pills is that they can both cause dementia and speed up existing dementias.

Finally, sleep apnea, a condition where a person's throat closes for very short amounts of time while sleeping, can cause a decrease of oxygen to the brain, which, in turn, can cause and worsen dementia. Sleep apnea improves significantly with a sleep apnea machine, called a CPAP—a mask that delivers a steady stream of pressurized air into the airway, keeping it open through the night. Many people resist CPAPs, especially dementia patients. They don't like masks. They don't like the sensation of air coming into their nasal and oral passageways. I don't think I would want that, either. Mom did have sleep apnea before and in the beginning of her Alzheimer's journey, which may have even contributed to her Alzheimer's. I tried, but she did not like the CPAC. Sleep apnea is correlated with being overweight. When Mom began her Alzheimer's journey and began her super healthy nutritional program, she lost enough unhealthy weight that her sleep apnea remarkably went away naturally. Today, there are a diversity of options for sleep apnea. If you see your loved one stop breathing for a moment and then coughing or gagging when sleeping, you are likely observing sleep apnea. Your loved one's PCP or sleep specialist doctor can help you diagnose this—there are machines available for home studies now—and decide if sleep apnea treatment makes sense.

Chapter Summary

1. Brain healthy nutrition is a very important pillar of the Breakthrough Care System. The brain, the body, and emotions (happiness) are linked systems that work together for a longer and happier life. Healthy nutrition plays a very important part in all three systems and can enhance your loved one's life in many ways. This chapter outlines Mom's healthy nutrition program and nutritional supplements that can fill any nutrition gaps due to swallowing or other concerns your loved one may have. Your doctor can help you modify the kind of nutrition program I describe here to fit your loved one's special needs.

2. Dementia patients often have swallowing issues. It is important that food be cut up finely, softened. or liquified. When a critically important brain healthy nutrient is not easily available in food form or cannot be swallowed safely by your loved one, find the most reputable companies for supplements. Also, find forms of taking them that are safer to swallow and better absorbed by the body (liquids and powders). Powders and liquids are easy to add to healthy and more easily swallowed food bases like soups, oatmeal, or smoothies.

3. Our wonderful caregivers made sure Mom ate and took all her pills, vitamins, and supplements safely and with great joy. They did this by watching Mom closely to make sure she was eating slowly and that her food was always cut up very finely. They also watched her swallow before taking another bite. They made mealtime fun and celebratory. This helped Mom be happy and more willing to eat and take her vitamins/supplements in the way her caregivers wanted.

    a. The complexity of the brain precludes proving the significance of a single nutrient. Consider using the suggested nutrients even if there may be only "some" or "limited" brain or body health evidence. Trusted versions can be found that are inexpensive and worth a try. Remember, many small benefits, including small nutritional benefits, can cumulatively help dementia patients in bigger breakthrough ways.

4. This chapter lists all the nutrition and supplements that helped Mom cognitively, physically, and emotionally. However, because the body often needs time to adjust and everyone is different, when trying a new nutritional ingredient, supplement, or medicine, I suggest starting with low doses and checking with your loved one's doctor and pharmacist. Your loved one's body may need time to get used to something new. It is better to go small and

very slowly than to risk a bad reaction and thereby losing the potential benefit of taking the supplement or medication at all.

5. Prescription medications and some supplements have both side effects and possible negative reactions on other aspects of your loved one's health. Make sure the benefits of one medication do not outweigh the harm it may cause to some other aspect of your loved one's health. Remember, elderly patients with dementia will have a different benefit/risk calculus than other patients. Involve your Alzheimer's specialist, neurologist, PCP, and pharmacist in helping you assess these tradeoffs for your loved one.

**Breakthrough Pillar #5
Fill Your Loved One's World
with Fun, Love, Compassion,
Stimulation, and Familiarity:
Physical Environment & People.**

All these things are key to dementia patients' happiness and cognitive health. Mom thrived when she was surrounded by people and a loving, familiar, stimulating, and fun environment. In these surroundings, you could see her face beam with joy and love. Mom's superpowered caregivers exuded these traits, but that was not enough for me. I wanted everything to reinforce all these things, all her people interactions, and her whole environment: all "touchpoints "needed to align and support these feelings in Mom at every moment of every day. All touchpoints had to be safe and exude love, positivity, familiarity, and stimulation. Like surround sound music, I wanted Mom to be surrounded by these things 24/7. An important care leader role is to design and maintain this ideal surround sound environment. By keeping Mom at home, I was able to design and ensure Mom's physical space and that all her people interactions created this desired environment with its associated benefits. If your loved one must be in a facility, you may not have full control, but I believe with empowered and active care leadership, it may be possible to influence the situation to create most of the breakthrough benefits of such a positively designed environment and people interactions.

CHAPTER 23

Surround Sound Physical Environment: A Consistently Fun, Familiar, Brain & Physically Stimulating Environment

Mom was surrounded by all the things she knew and loved, which meant she stayed engaged, comfortable, and positive. This, in turn, made her happier, confident, and less stressed through her Alzheimer's journey. Everyone likes the familiar and being around things they know and love. This is especially true if you are scared. I can't imagine anything scarier than what dementia patients go through, very slowly losing your memory, losing the people you love, losing the things you know and do, and losing who you are. Surrounding your loved one with all the things that they love and are familiar with is very important for reducing this fear. We decided to keep Mom in her same room at home with all her familiar keepsakes. As Mom's Alzheimer's progressed, the only thing that we changed was to make her environment safer, without giving up anything familiar or comforting. As mentioned in the safety chapter, we put the half bed rails on her bed and then covered these bed rails with her favorite-colored Afghans. By making the bed look more welcoming and homier, we both made Mom feel more comfortable and kept her skin safe from sharp rail edges. Another example of safety while not compromising familiarity and fun is decorating her walker and her wheelchair with familiar items like her dolls, stuffed animals, and ribbons that made Mom feel comfortable and familiar when we went out on our daily adventures. These again were intended to make Mom feel warm and secure and to have fun with all aspects of her experience.

We kept all Mom's photos, dolls, stuffed animals, and, of course, her Betty Boop collection in her bedroom. We always decorated the house with balloons, tableware, favors, and cakes to reflect each holiday. Mom loved all the holidays and used to decorate the house so festively for all our birthdays and holidays. When she taught kindergarten, she always decorated the classroom with all kinds of holiday fun items and kids' drawings. You could really see that Mom's kindergarteners had lots of fun and did many creative activities in the classroom. We tried to keep that same fun spirit and creativity alive with Mom at home every single day.

We played music and sang songs Mom loved. Because Mom loved clothing styles all her life, our caregivers always had a new fashion magazine for her to thumb through and enjoy. Also, we placed the pictures that Mom drew around the house because we wanted to send a message to her that we loved her very much, that the art she created was important to us, and that we were proud of her (just like you would do for your child). Our house was a fun place to live because it was filled with festive and familiar things for Mom. For Mom's entire journey, we helped dress her in the morning every day, in regular clothes (not her nighttime PJs), so she would be comfortable and happy with beautiful clothes that were familiar to her. Getting dressed is what she did every day of her life, so continuing that familiar and comforting routine was important. Mom's caregivers always let her choose what she wanted to wear each day. Empowering her to choose was also very good for Mom. She loved her stylish clothing and kept her "fine" clothing most of her life. Mom could not speak, but she would point out what shirt or skirt that she wanted to wear. Our wonderful caregivers would always make sure Mom wore the outfit she wanted. She loved to look "spruced up," stylish, and pretty; her caregivers would put lipstick and makeup on her every day. They would look in the mirror together, and Mom would laugh, make faces at her caregiver, and admire her look and the makeup. Her caregivers not only used these make-up sessions as a chance for Mom to participate in the familiar routine she had before Alzheimer's but also to maintain her pride and self-esteem.

Everything about Mom's surround sound environment was designed to keep things familiar, like her past, with as much fun and love as possible. Mom loved the home that she created for our family, and she worked very hard to keep us safe and happy as we grew up. She had much pride and love in every beautiful household effect and treasure that she added to our home. We wanted to keep those memories and positive feelings in her home front and center for her every day.

Our home and the treasures that Mom chose for us are beautiful memories for us, too. Why in the world would we want to change any of that? The more her daily environment included the same surround-sound of love, familiarity and fun, the better. We were successful in adding safety without taking away any of the love, fun, familiarity, and comfort that had always been there. The last thing we wanted for Mom was the sterile environment of some hospitals, nursing homes, and other care facilities. You'll want your loved one's surroundings to reflect as much as possible the familiar love and warmth they knew best. Even if your loved one is in a facility, help make that environment fun, familiar, comforting, and stimulating. Your loved one will be much happier if you do.

CHAPTER 24

Surround Sound People Environment: Fun, Familiar, Creatively Comforting, Stimulating, Compassionate, and Loving People Only

In addition to Mom's physical environment being a surround sound of comfort, familiarity, and fun, I wanted every single person who encountered Mom every day to reflect the same. As discussed, I carefully selected caregivers with the skills to reflect the behaviors of fun, positive and creative stimulation, comfort, and love. I also regularly encouraged, recognized, and reinforced these behaviors. I worked to create the positive and flexible environment to keep Mom's remarkable caregivers so long that they became part of our family, a loving, fun, and enduring family for Mom. As Mom spent time with our new caregiver extended family, Marina, and me, she deeply enjoyed her experiences every single day and night.

Early in our journey, when I was still learning about what good caregiving was all about, I saw a caregiver impatiently correcting Mom a lot. When I observed this, the hairs went up on the back of my neck because I could see Mom starting to lose her champion smile. She seemed very uncomfortable with that caregiver. When Marina and I were growing up, our mom rarely criticized or corrected us in any negative way. We always felt supported and loved and had a lot of fun with Mom. I did not want a critical and impatient caregiver or anyone else she encountered to create a negative or sad environment for Mom, especially when she now needed to be loved and have more positivity and fun than ever.

I have heard many people share how devastated they were when their loved ones could not remember them. Because some people can't tolerate that kind of heartache, they may be tempted to visit or be with them less often. We were very fortunate because my mom did remember us for her entire Alzheimer's journey. It probably helped that we lived together at home and saw each other every day. I observed that if someone came every day or at least every 12-14 days Mom would know who they were. If someone came less often than that, Mom would usually not remember who they were. Our wonderful caregivers would see Mom nearly every day. Her physical therapist came once a week, so Mom knew him. As you carefully observe your loved one, you might see a version of this kind of recognition pattern. You may need to adjust your visiting schedule or others' visiting schedules to fit your loved one's memory. Seeing people who come often enough to be remembered can enhance your loved one's joy at seeing them. Your loved one's visitors, care providers, or therapists, I'm sure, will enjoy being recognized, too, likely improving the positivity and effectiveness of each of their interactions with your loved one.

The more your loved one is surrounded and touched by people every day who are full of love, creative, caring, and fun the better. Whether your loved one is in a facility or at home if the caregivers keep changing, even if they are fun and loving, your loved one will not feel loved and safe because these individuals are not familiar to them. Think about this as you reflect on who visits your loved one, regardless of whether they are friends, family, or professionals. As care leader, encourage family, friends, and professionals to always reflect these supportive traits and to visit regularly. The more regular the visit, the more familiar the caregiver will be to your loved one and therefore the more supportive and beneficial the interaction. Even if it is difficult and sad to see your loved one declining, be positive, fun, and compassionately loving. Your loved one needs that positivity from you, your caregivers, friends, and professionals in every single interaction every single day. Your planning for and protecting these interactions will be rewarded tenfold with your loved one's greater peace and joy!

As Mom's care leader I saw that one of my important jobs was to create and protect her environment and her experiences. I wanted every physical, environmental, and people touchpoint to reflect the Breakthrough Care System traits. If a care provider, therapist, or other specialist coming to the house, or anyone visiting did not reflect these traits, I did not want them near Mom. Anyone projecting criticism, negativity, impatience, or frustration with Mom or mom's behavior had to go. This was too important not to have high expectations for her environment and every interaction.

Planning and nurturing Mom's entire surround sound experience led to Mom's difficult Alzheimer's journey being that much smoother and happier. I believe this environment contributed to Mom's greater longevity. Happier people want to live longer—and often do.

Summary

1. Be thoughtful about your loved one's daily physical environment and interactions. If they are surrounded by all the things they are used to, have creative and stimulating fun, and feel compassionately loved and cherished, they will feel happier and more like their old selves. If your loved one's environment is too sterile, bring in as many of the things they love and are fun to them as you can.

2. Every person who touches your loved one every single day must be fun, loving, caring, stimulating, and familiar to your loved one. If any person that comes to see your loved one is impatient, critical, or does not positively engage with them in a loving way, either make sure they don't come back or coach them in their behavior.

3. If caregivers or other care specialists coming to see your loved one are constantly changing or do not exhibit the Breakthrough Care System traits, your loved one's self-esteem and sense of security will falter. It is better to have those who see your loved

one come at the same time/day if possible; dementia patients need structure, regularity, and routine to feel comfortable and safe. If people who see your loved one don't come frequently and regularly, your loved one likely won't recognize them and therefore more likely to be agitated and anxious.

4. I encourage you to consider that one of your very important overall care leader roles is to be your loved one's "Experience Designer and Protector" (a fancy title, I know). If your loved one's physical environment and the people who come in to contact with your loved one do not consistently and completely reflect and reinforce these desired "surround sound" feelings and experiences your loved one will not be as happy, positively stimulated, comforted or safe as is necessary for breakthrough results in longevity and happiness. Think of your new role of "Experience Designer and Protector" as a creative exercise of love for your loved one.

Medical Mistakes: Tragically Cutting a Long Alzheimer's Journey Short

CHAPTER 25

Decision-Making Errors
When Tired and under Stress

In this love story so far, Mom has flourished beautifully. I have tried to show what it takes to be a strong and empowered breakthrough care leader. I know since I was able to be this empowered care leader, you will be one, too. I am about to bring what may be a relatively positive image of me crashing back to earth. I made an error in judgement (that I want you to avoid), and that error led to a great deal of pain and suffering for Mom. What I describe in this chapter is by far the biggest mistake in my life. I regret it deeply. I share it to help you avoid it.

On Friday January 6, 2020, Mom woke up and was not her usual smiling and happy self. Something was very wrong. Over the course of the day, Paula, Marina, and I grew worried. We took Mom's oxygen saturation level and blood pressure. Her oxygen saturation level was low, and her heart rate was fast. Mom seemed short of breath, and she was very tired. After a little while, I called Mom's PCP and told her Mom's symptoms and vitals. She suggested we take her to the Emergency Room.

We packed Mom up and drove her there. After a few tests, the ER doctor told me she was suffering from a touch of congestive heart failure. They wanted to check her into a room on the Cardiac Floor for observation and additional tests. This was just before the pandemic hit so we were able to go in with Mom. As they wheeled Mom into her room, we all held her hand. One of her stuffed animals was on her chest. I looked into Mom's eyes, and I could see she was scared. This frightened me because Mom never acted afraid. Her room-lighting smile was gone.

Once we checked her into her room, we tried to make things as comfortable and as familiar as we could. A hospital is a scary and unfamiliar place for anyone, especially an Alzheimer's patient. We knew it would be nearly impossible to make this hospital room exactly like her familiar room at home, but we tried. Marina went home and picked up many of Mom's stuffed animals, cozy blankets, a Betty Boop doll, flowers, and some other things Mom loved and scattered them about the hospital room. We brought magazines that Mom liked to thumb through and her coloring books and pencils. The nurses were nice to allow us to transform this sterile hospital room into a much warmer and more familiar place for Mom.

I spoke to the hospitalist assigned to my mom, and he told me what medications she would get and about some of the tests they were going to do. I told him that Mom had Alzheimer's and what medications she was currently taking. He ordered the cardiac medications and her regular prescription medicines. He, unfortunately, was not able provide the non-prescription nutrient supplements for Mom and told us that Mom would probably be in the hospital for at least a couple of days. I thought for a couple of days it would probably be okay for Mom not to take them.

Like all hospitals, the noise and activities began in and outside her room. Poor Mom! They hooked her up to all kinds of monitors and IVs. Blood and other tests had started and were getting more frequent. I saw in Mom's face that she was trying to be her usual cooperative and happy self, but I could also see she was very scared, annoyed, and disoriented. I knew I needed to be there as much as possible to keep her comfortable and calm and to be her advocate and decision maker.

Alzheimer's patients and many elderly patients need a family member to advocate for them with doctors and hospitals. I knew I needed and wanted to be in this room with her 24 hours a day until she left. I texted all of Mom's remarkable caregivers and told them that Mom was in the hospital and that I wasn't sure whether Mom needed them in the hospital or even whether they wanted to come to the hospital to help her. They all immediately said they wanted to come and be there for Mom, Marina, and me. Each ended up working their regular shift with Mom in her hospital room. I was happy because I knew they would help create a more normal and regular environment for Mom and would allow me to focus on Mom's medical care while I was there. The nurses were very good about allowing Mom's caregivers and me in the room at the same time. I really appreciated that.

The cardiac floor had good nurses and pretty good patient coverage. However, even here, nurses were not always available when Mom needed care. Mom's super caregivers really filled that gap, physically and emotionally, and helped her have as much fun as possible, given her condition and being in a hospital. They helped the nurses with cleaning Mom, getting her in and out of bed, observing and rotating her so she would not get bed sores and other very important, non-medical, aspects of care. Just as important, our caregivers knew how to make Mom feel comfortable and a little more like her happier self. With their help, I was able to get a couple of hours of sleep overnight on the little fold-up bed provided in Mom's room. I was immensely grateful for our caregivers; they were truly a gift to us in so many ways.

The hospitalist, who was very nice and had good awareness of Mom's condition and progress, indulged the stream of questions that I would ask him several times a day. Moreover, I was able to obtain the daily records of all the tests, medications, and various fluids and nutrition given to my mom.

After a couple of days, Mom's heart tests started to show improvement. However, the hospitalist told me that Mom seemed to have some trouble breathing and her oxygen level had declined some, about which the staff was concerned. Mom's regular (non-guru) local pulmonologist came to visit Mom. After taking an x-ray and listening to her lungs, he said she had contracted pneumonia in the hospital. Unfortunately, this is one of the common risks of being in a hospital. Being in bed makes elderly patients prone to pneumonia. It is also very easy to get a pneumonia virus from the staff or other patients in a hospital setting. As her heart became better, Mom was moved to a regular (non-cardiac floor) room. We took all Mom's familiar home decorations and redecorated her new hospital room. Mom was given antibiotics, nebulizer treatments, and shaking-the-lungs treatments for her pneumonia. With a touch of congestive heart failure and now pneumonia, Mom had become very weak. After another week in the hospital, Mom's vitals improved, yet, understandably, she was still very wan and very tired. Because of this and probably also because Mom was not in her comfortable home environment, she stopped eating. The hospitalist shared with me his worry about her not eating, noting that she needed nutrition to continue to get stronger and better.

The hospitalist outlined three choices. The staff was optimistic that Mom might be discharged in a few days, but the eating issue needed to be addressed.

One choice was to feed Mom intravenously—a short-term solution because long-term IV nutrition can lead to blood clotting and her important prescription medicines could not be compounded and given through IV. IV feeding, though, if chosen as the approach to use, could continue when she went home or to a rehab facility but would require skilled nursing help.

The second option, a gastrostomy (feeding) tube, or G-tube, could be surgically implanted in Mom's stomach for feeding. Her crushed prescription pills and her liquid and powder supplements could be given through the G-tube. Feeding through the G-tube could be continued at home, without skilled nursing, relatively easily by our caregivers or by me. When Mom regained her strength and started eating real food, we could take her back to the hospital as an outpatient and the G-tube could be easily removed. The hospitalist told me that implantation of a G-tube was a routine and safe procedure.

The third option was to discharge Mom when she was ready and hope that at home she would be more comfortable and quickly begin eating. If she did not begin eating right away at home, we could always take her back into the hospital for implantation of a G-tube.

I had an important decision to make, but I did not have much time to make it. It was urgent because Mom needed nutrition now. As a former human resources person, I have taught leaders about decision making. One of the tools I taught leaders to use to make important decisions is a decision matrix. The way a decision matrix works is you put your values or what's most important to you on one side of the matrix with a numerical weighting (like 1-5) of how important each value is to you. Then, on the other side of the matrix, you list the decision choices. After that, you select a number (like 1-5) that estimates how well each decision achieves each of the important values you listed. Then, you add those numbers together for each choice and see which option has the largest number. By doing this you get a quantitative snapshot of which decision is better in meeting what's important to you.

Given the importance of the decision, I thought the decision matrix might help, so I started creating a matrix. To collect data, I quickly called a couple of physicians on Mom's team for their opinion. Mom's PCP said the G-tube was low risk and might really help. I called my own PCP who thought bringing Mom home to see if she would start eating would probably be better. Mom's neurologist thought the IV nutrition might be a good first step as it was a little less invasive than a G-tube, could get Mom some nutrition, and would buy a little time until she started eating at home. After hearing each of these disparate views, I did my own internet search on G-tubes, and IV nutrition to complete the decision matrix.

A Black Swan Event in Decision Making

Considering the pros and cons to all three options, I was leaning toward the G-tube, but before I decided, I wanted to speak briefly with the surgeon who would do the procedure. Mom had never had the need for this kind of surgeon and there was no time to find and bring in a "stomach surgeon guru." I was dependent on the hospital's assignment of surgeon. The procedure was supposed to be easy and routine, so they sent a surgeon up to the floor who had experience with laparoscopic stomach surgeries. He assured me that this was a simple, routine surgical implant and my mom would do just fine. To be sure there would be no surprises, the surgeon wanted to do a quick stomach scan first. After viewing the scan, the surgeon refused to place a G-tube because apparently Mom had a tremendous amount of scar tissue in the area of her stomach. My sister remembered that Mom had had gallbladder surgery in her twenties and that apparently was the source of the scar tissue. The surgeon said that he could not place a G-tube because the scar tissue would not only make the operation too dangerous but also would potentially reject the G-tube, most likely causing an infection. He doubted that the G- tube could be adequately anchored in the stomach. Instead of a G-tube, he recommended a J-Tube (Jejunostomy), a feeding tube placed lower in the intestine, avoiding the scar tissue. Mom would have the benefits of a G-tube without the risks of infection and rejection.

After reviewing the options and the decision matrix, I told the surgeon to go forward with the J-tube. He scheduled the surgery for the next day. Though everyone said this kind of feeding tube was routine and very safe, for some reason my intuition told me that something was wrong. I called our church and asked that one of our priests come to the hospital and give Mom the Anointing of the Sick sacrament and Apostolic Pardon blessing. These are special graces for forgiveness of sins that a priest can provide when someone is at risk of passing. One of our wonderful parish priests, Father Thomas, came out immediately and gave these to Mom. I was very grateful for his kind and uplifting spirit and to our Parish for enabling him to come quickly to see Mom.

Everyone said I should not be nervous about the routine J-tube procedure, yet I was. A voice in my head told me to write a note in Mom's medical chart confirming that the doctor was doing a J-tube and not a G-tube and the reason why. I wrote the note and gave it to the hospitalist, asking him to make sure it was in Mom's medical chart for the surgical team to see prior to the surgery. The hospitalist said he didn't deem this necessary but would do it anyway.

Mom immediately went into surgery and after a while came out of recovery. Then, they wheeled her back to her room. Mom's face was sad, and she looked even more scared than before. I looked down at the feeding tube. I know where the stomach is, and this feeding tube was protruding out of Mom's stomach, not her intestine. I felt shocked, confused, and worried! I asked the nurse about this; she looked at Mom's stomach and confirmed that this was a G-tube. I was perplexed. The surgeon specifically said he would not do the G-tube because of the risks involved. What in the world was going on here?

Within 24 hours, the skin around the G-tube had turned bright red and started to ooze black gunk. Mom quickly developed a fever, and her nurse said she did not like the look of the stomach wound site where the G-tube was inserted. By the next morning, it looked horrible. A tremendous amount of black ooze was coming out of the hole where the G-tube had been inserted. Mom's entire stomach blistered bright red with a major infection. The hospital's infectious disease doctor put Mom on super strong antibiotics. Two days later, the infection had worsened. The amount of oozing black coming out of the stomach hole was greater, and the skin redness had spread to her back. The doctor added pain and high-fever medications. Mom was clearly in pain and very scared, but as always, she was acting bravely for us. When I was growing up, Mom was always brave for us. She always tried to make things easy and good for Marina and me. I was proud of her courage, but I also was very worried and confused about what was happening. I took photos several times a day of this horrible infection and sent them to the hospitalist. The surgeon would not return my calls to explain why he put in the G-tube instead of the agreed upon J-tube. The hospitalist either did not know or would not tell me.

Every day the infection and fever worsened. The infectious disease doctor changed Mom's medication to a different, even stronger antibiotic. All the nurses on this surgical floor told us that they had never seen an infection this bad. At about this time, like a cork, the whole feeding tube just popped out of Mom's stomach. That's right…the feeding tube popped out! The nurses said they had never seen a feeding tube pop out like that. Like the surgeon warned, the scar tissue apparently rejected the tube. My head was spinning. I kept thinking, "Why did the surgeon do the very procedure that he said would be so dangerous?" I asked everybody, and nobody could—or would—give me an answer!

Because the G-tube came out, Mom was taken to a special Lab for insertion of an IV feeding line so she could at least get some hydration, nutrition, and medication. Mom suffered in this infectious state for two weeks, with constant changes to prescribed antibiotics, but nothing ameliorated the rampant infection. Every day I would tell anyone who would listen that something had to be done!!! Mom's fever was still very high, and I could see her fading, slowly dying in front of me! The staff iced her down continuously to reduce her fever, and the doctors kept changing her antibiotics. Nothing was working. Things were very bad. Finally, the doctors decided they had no choice but to operate again and surgically remove all the horrible black infection and ooze that was now growing everywhere inside of her. I knew that surgery of this nature had to be a big, long, and very risky procedure, which is I'm sure why they delayed so long to do it. I saw no choice because Mom's life was on the line now. She would have died very soon if something wasn't done. I reluctantly agreed, and Mom went back into surgery.

This surgery, especially given Mom's age and frail Alzheimer's condition was super risky. It was very long and very difficult. Mom was in surgery for almost five hours. I was petrified as to whether she would survive the surgery and what her cognitive state would be if she did. When Mom, with God's grace, came out of surgery, the surgical wound was completely covered. Later, the nurse removed the bandages to clean the wound and change the dressing. I have a very strong stomach, but the first time I saw the open wound I almost threw up. The nurse measured it. The wound along her stomach was 15 inches long, five inches wide, and four inches deep. I could see the entire inside of Mom's stomach area. I asked why it was not sewn up. The wound care nurse said that the size and depth of the wound made it too large to sew up. They thought a wound vac machine would keep the wound dry and help the healing. Mom's touch of congestive heart failure and pneumonia had improved after about two weeks. However, with this feeding tube horror, the resultant infection, the delayed surgery to remove the infection and infected tissue, and now time needed for healing, Mom had been in the hospital for nearly eight weeks. My wonderful and loving Mom was suffering tremendously from the botched-up feeding tube fiasco caused by botched-up actions of the surgeon. What a nightmare!!! I was very angry and very scared.

The more I thought about it, the angrier I got!! I laid on the rollout bed in Mom's hospital room and stared at the ceiling, thinking how we had worked so hard for so long to keep Mom out of a hospital and then this idiot surgeon's mistake had created a nightmare I could not even imagine. This "simple, routine, and safe" feeding tube procedure had turned into a monstrous horror. I kept wondering, "What happened and where did I go wrong as Mom's care leader?" Doing the wrong feeding tube procedure in the exact wrong place was a "Black Swan Event." The term comes from the financial world as an event that is impossible to predict. Who could have predicted that a surgeon could do the wrong procedure in the wrong place? He turned a safe and simple procedure into an unimaginable nightmare threatening my loving Mom's life.

I was incredibly upset. I tried again to ask the surgeon how this happened. Neither he nor anyone else would talk to me. The president of the hospital would not take my calls, so I wrote a letter to him. I received no response. I quickly filed a formal complaint with the hospital review committee. A few days later, they said they had received the complaint but could not talk about it. In fact, I never heard anything back from any of these people or from the hospital review committee.

You cannot predict this kind of horrible event for your loved one, but in retrospect I should have brought Mom home and trusted she would have started eating again. With the stress and exhaustion of being at the hospital 24/7, I think I panicked and forgot how strong Mom was and how much she loved being home. I also forgot how talented her remarkable caregivers were and the beautiful connection they had with Mom. They would have found a way to get Mom to eat again. I completely underestimated Mom and our wonderful caregivers. I was feeling so down about myself and my decision I started crying uncontrollably in that little hospital room. My decision to do the feeding tube made sense to me at the time, but I was dead wrong! At that moment, staring at the ceiling in Mom's hospital room, I felt like a huge failure as a care leader and as a son. I was very deep in the basement on the mood elevator.

After more than ten weeks in the hospital, with daily wound care, wound vac machines, and lots more very strong antibiotics and pain medications, the Grand Canyon-sized open surgical wound was beginning to shrink, and the fever was getting better. Thank you, God!! Mom's wonderful caregivers stayed with me in the hospital room 24/7 the whole time. They, along with wonderful nurses, took beautiful care of Mom. Our caregivers helped me be more positive and helped pulled me out of my self-blame and depression. I prayed many times a day; I would leave the hospital room for a bit to pray in the hospital chapel, soak in a moment of sunshine, or grab a quick snack before going back to the hospital room to be with Mom. Even though, like Mom, I had a giant hole inside of me, I knew I had to stay strong for Mom and for Marina. I was always grateful for our loving caregivers but never so much as I was during the depths of my depression after this feeding tube disaster.

There is no doubt that my wonderful grandmother would have called this stomach surgeon a shoemaker (or worse). I am very grateful that I did not see this shoemaker in the hospital cafeteria when I went for a quick snack. I don't know what I would have done if I had seen him, but I know it would not have been good for him or for me.

After a few more days the hospitalist told me that Mom was well enough that she could soon leave the hospital for a rehab facility for continued wound vac care, IV feeding, and physical therapy. Given that Mom and I had been living in this hospital for eleven weeks and because in this hospital she had gotten both pneumonia and a botched-up death-threatening surgery, I knew she was not going to another facility.

I ambulanced Mom home. I have never been so happy to see our wonderful house the day we took Mom home. It was like heaven to see the overgrown front yard, the house's old paint, and the repairs I've had to put off. Our neighbors welcomed us home. We were so happy.

This was March 2020. Even though I knew this time home care would be much tougher, it was the right thing to do. Mom's survival was a gift from God. All the medical equipment was delivered, and the nursing visits were scheduled. The nurses came and taught our caregivers and me how to do the IV feeding, put antibiotics in the IV system, and operate the wound vac machine. They checked on Mom, on us, and the equipment, put in new IV lines, and did the surgical wound dressing changes. These hospital nurses were terrific—very compassionate and nice. The hospital also sent a physician to see Mom once a week. This at-home physician was also very compassionate and competent. I was so happy we could do everything at home that would have been done in a rehab facility. Mom was surrounded by all the people she loved and who loved her. Even though things were still so very hard for Mom, I saw a happy little glint in Mom's eye and even a glimpse of her room -lighting smile. I could tell Mom was happy to be out of the hospital and at home.

Mom came home just in time because this was the very beginning of the first COVID wave. Many people were blocked from seeing their loved ones in hospitals and other facilities during COVID. At home, we wore masks and made sure caregivers, nurses, and therapists were regularly tested for COVID. This was a minor inconvenience; if Mom had been in a facility, it would have been horrible because we likely would not have been able to be with her.

The hospital also sent physical and occupational therapists regularly to get Mom out of bed and moving again. Mom slowly began to eat a little soft food and drink along with her IV nutrition. The huge surgical wound monster very slowly was healing. After a little more than month at home, the four months of super strong IV antibiotics were finally discontinued. Mom was more alert and started to smile again and interact with our caregivers, Marina, and me. Mom's congestive heart failure and pneumonia were completely gone. Mom was starting to eat a little more and take her pills and supplements again. After about five weeks at home, things finally appeared to be looking up. I felt so blessed and grateful!

Chapter Summary

1. Even in a hospital, you can create a surrounding environment of fun, familiarity, stimulation, and love. Within limits, you can decorate a hospital room like a room at home. Hospital nurses are busy and focused more on medical care; bringing your regular home or private caregivers to the hospital can be done and will have a tremendous value to your loved one and to you.

2. As a reminder, when a doctor says something is routine and safe, they may be speaking from their general experience. Your loved one may not fit the averages. Just be cautious when you hear "it's easy, safe, and routine" from a physician. Any invasive procedure can be life threatening for an elderly patient. Really consider the most conservative treatment first. There is usually time to do the more invasive solution later if the conservative one does not work.

3. Any surgery can be dangerous. If your loved one must have it, take the extra time to get the best surgeon possible. If possible, don't just automatically take the surgeon that the hospital assigns. Research the surgeon to be sure there are no malpractice claims or other infractions against the doctor (tips on how to do this are in the Resources Section). Medical mistakes and malpractice are far more common than anyone knows. Please, don't allow shoemaker surgeons, like I did, to take care of your loved one.

4. If your loved one is in the hospital for something serious and needs complex rehab when they are discharged, you can do all this rehab (even with complex equipment and skilled nursing requirements) at home. Recall there is nothing, including doctors, that you can get in a rehab facility that you cannot get in the comfort and familiarity of your home.

I am encouraged to think that, if this ever happened to your loved one and you, by learning from my horrific experience, you would not make the same mistake of being too aggressive in medical treatment. Yes, the surgeon made a grievous mistake that no one could have predicted, but I should have been more conservative. I believe with the elderly, and especially elderly dementia patients, unless your loved one's life is in immediate jeopardy without surgery, it is better to be more conservative in treatment. I should have taken a more conservative approach and trusted Mom would eat at home. She ended up eating at home, but not until she had undergone more unnecessary suffering than anyone should have to bear. It is one of the biggest mistakes I have made in my whole life. I am hopeful you will learn this from our nightmare.

CHAPTER 26

Black Swan Gets Blacker

After that marathon hospital stay, Mom continued to gain strength at home. She began walking again; her wonderful smiling and loving self was slowly coming back. Then, one day the Black Swan tragic medical mistake raised its ugly head. It was May 2020, nearly three months after Mom arrived back home; Luisa who had been with Mom overnight reported to me that she did not like the way Mom was breathing. Alma was just coming on in the morning, and we took Mom's vitals. Mom's heartbeat was very rapid, her blood pressure was low, and her temperature was high. She also had very bad diarrhea, and her oxygen saturation was low. I called the physician who had been coming to our house weekly. She wanted me to take Mom to the Emergency Room. You could imagine after the disaster of such a long hospital stay just two months ago, I was not eager to return Mom to the hospital. I decided to wait a bit and continue to evaluate Mom. I waited until that afternoon. We took her vitals again, and they were not good at all. I could tell Mom was struggling. It went against every fiber of my being to take her to that hospital again, but I did. I called the ambulance. I was scared to death and started praying harder than ever.

They took Mom into the ER for testing. This was May 2020, and the first wave of Covid had hit hard. I was unable to go into the ER with Mom. I had to wait for the doctor outside for what seemed like forever. The doctor finally came out. The first thing he asked me was if it would be okay, if necessary, to put Mom on a ventilator. He also asked me end-of-life decisions. I thought to myself, "This is not good!" I said I had decision-making authority for all end-of-life things and wanted him to do everything possible to keep Mom alive. The ER doctor said Mom's lungs were not working right, but he was not sure why. He said Mom needed to be checked into the Intensive Care Unit (ICU). Then, he said because of Covid I had to go home. I told him that with her Alzheimer's Mom could not speak for herself and would be scared and very disoriented. I told him I understood about Covid rules but needed to be with her. I told him that, if necessary, I would wear a mask, a gown, or a space suit if that's what it took to stay with her. He said he was sorry, but these were the rules: no family or guests of any kind. I went home very frustrated, upset, and scared!

Rock Stars, Sisters, And Thinking Outside the Box

When I got home, I told my sister Marina what was going on. She knew how important it was to be there with Mom in the hospital. She, too, was very frustrated we couldn't be with her. Then, Marina anxiously blurted, "Call the President and get an exception so we can see Mom!"

Surprised, I asked her, "what President?"

She replied, "Call the President of the United States, Donald Trump!"

"What?" I responded, "Donald Trump? Really?"

My overly practical experience working in a company kicked in. I told her, "We can't call Trump!"

Regardless, I found an email address for Donald Trump and emailed him our request. We waited about 30 minutes, Surprise, we did not hear back from President Trump.

Then in my sister's awesome, but powerfully naïve way, she blurted out again, "Then call the mayor and ask for an exception!"

I told her that I had never spoken to our mayor, either. Because we felt so desperate, I called the mayor's office anyway. We *were* desperate. A caring, wonderfully sweet elderly woman answered the mayor's phone. I explained to her what was going on and that we desperately needed to be with our mom in the hospital. She told me that the mayor and the entire city council was in a meeting at the city library to talk, ironically, about COVID. She said that if I emailed them all right now, since they were together, some or all of them might see the request at the same time. I quickly went online to the city website and found the council members' and mayor's email addresses and composed the email request. I wrote about how serious Mom's condition was, about her Alzheimer's, and about how much our mom needed us to be there to be her advocate, decision maker, and comfort.

Ten minutes after launching the email, a true Christmas-in-May miracle happened! I received an email back from one of the council members. The councilwoman, Diane Dixon, said she knew a senior leader at the hospital. Her email said there were no guarantees, but she would see what she could do.

After another five minutes, I received a follow-up email from her. It said that I should go to the hospital and provide my name. I would then be able to see Mom, but only one family member would be allowed in the hospital.

At that moment, I had so much respect for my naïve, bold, and genius of a sister! I thought her idea to call the mayor was silly, but she is a genius. My grandmother was talking to her, "Where there is a will, there is a way!" I would never have thought of calling the mayor or city council. I thought I was creative and tenacious, but Marina was the role model for determination and bold thinking outside the bun that day! Maybe Marina was also channeling Winston Churchill during the depths of World War II who so famously said "Never, never, never, never give up," or maybe she inherited that trait from our creative and delightfully determined mother.

I immediately drove to the hospital. A very long line of family and guests were trying to talk their way into the hospital. All were very upset and angry that they could not get into the hospital to see their loved ones. I passed the angry mob and stood in the front of the line. I gave my name, and they took my temperature and made sure I was wearing a mask. Then, they waved me in.

I felt strangely guilty yet very happy that I had just strolled right in front of everybody in line and gone in. It could not have been any easier. People waiting in line must have thought I was a rock star or celebrity. I've been to a few rock concerts, but I don't think that gives me rock star credentials. To my amazement I later found out that this rock star pass into the hospital was not just a one-time pass but a pass to go into and out of the hospital any time I wanted for as long as Mom was there!! Wow! Diane Dixon had given me big time celebrity credentials! I thought, "Thank you so much, Diane," and I thought, "Move over Mick Jagger, there is a new rock star in town."

When I walked into the hospital lobby that COVID day for the first time, it was truly a ghost town. I was the only guest or family member that I could see in the entire hospital. The hospital appeared completely empty. I saw a couple of nurses, but that was all. It starkly contrasted with the business and craziness of the hospital a couple of months ago when I had been literally living there for months with Mom. God bless my bold and wonderful sister, and God bless the bold and wonderful Diane Dixon, too.[3] I will be forever grateful to her.

Covid Time, Loneliness, and God's Grace

I found Mom's room in the ICU. I sat with her. We held hands. As I held her hand, for some reason memories started streaming uncontrollably into my brain. I remembered that Mom was always very affectionate and loving. She loved to hug and kiss us. When Mom smiled, all the world's troubles would fade. She took such amazingly good care of Marina and me for so very long. Mom made our world wonderful and fun. Mom always helped me with schoolwork. She defended me no matter what trouble I was in. Now I must fight for and defend her with every power I could muster. Looking at Mom in the ICU and seeing how bad she looked, I felt horrible. There was no smile, and I felt so bad that I could hardly breathe myself.

---

3. As a side note, this terrific councilwoman, who helped us so much in our darkest hour, later ran for State Assembly. I owed her so much for getting me in to see Mom that I happily helped her campaign for the assembly seat, and she won! Good things happen to good people!

The BiPAP machine, which delivers pressurized air through a mask to support breathing, was no longer sufficient. To ensure adequate oxygenation, they transitioned her to a ventilator, intubating her (placing a tube into her trachea) to assist her breathing more directly. Seeing Mom on a ventilator broke my heart.

After a few hours, the doctor came in and explained that they did tests and found that Mom had c. diff and sepsis. I knew c. diff was mostly caused by taking too many strong antibiotics for too long. Because of the medical mistake by the idiot stomach surgeon, Mom had to be on very strong IV antibiotics for four months. These antibiotics had to have caused her c. diff. Sepsis also follows bad infections and c. diff, especially in patients like Mom who are weakened or immuno-compromised. It was two days before Mother's Day, and now c. diff and the accompanying sepsis was Mom's glorious Mother's Day gift from her surgeon. Once again, thank you, you (expletive) shoemaker doctor!! The Black Swan was quickly getting blacker.

I sat next to Mom, who was on the ventilator. I sat with her, holding her hand. I thought Mom was the bravest and strongest person I have ever known. Late the first night when I was holding Mom's hand in the ICU, it was eerily quiet, sad, and lonely. The ICU nurses offered me a rollaway and treated me very nicely. Even though I was the only privileged guest in the entire hospital that night, they all knew I was not Mick Jagger or any other rock star. How did they know that? First, I do not have a British accent, and second, rock stars are usually rowdy and rambunctious. I was not; I am sure I looked like the saddest person on the planet at that moment. I sat there, feeling very lonely, sad, angry, scared, and upset in my yellow COVID sanitary gown and mask.

My mind toggled between praying to God for help and reflecting on my decision to do that stupid feeding tube that directly led to all this suffering. I kept getting stuck in my thinking: "If I had brought Mom home from the hospital right after her pneumonia improved, she would have started eating again when she got home." Bringing Mom home with IV nutrition and then transitioning to real food would have been so much better. That, after all, is what she ended up doing, anyway. I thought, "How could I have let this happen? How could I have been so stupid?" I felt profoundly guilty that my decision had caused so much suffering for the most wonderful woman, teacher, and mom who ever existed. I could not help obsessing again!! Of course, hindsight is always 20/20, but I could not get this horrible sense of blame out of my head!!

After I snapped myself out of this obsessively depressed daze, all I could hear was the constant thumping sound of Mom's ventilator. I got up to turn on Mom's TV and found a channel that played some Disney movies. Mom loved to watch Disney movies. I've heard that when someone is in a light coma like Mom was, they can hear. I didn't know if Mom might hear it or like it, but, just in case, I put on the Disney movie *Frozen*, which she loved, and tried to get my mind off the botched-up surgery and my botched-up decision making. Seeing Mom breathe with this machine and with tubes coming out of every orifice was worse than the worst horror movie I have ever seen. In the dead quiet of the middle of the night, staring at this horrible ventilator monster, I suddenly jumped up the mood elevator. I thought, "Mom recovered from congestive heart failure, hospital-acquired pneumonia, a horrible stomach surgery mistake, infection, and a Grand Canyon-sized stomach surgery wound. If she got through all these things, then she is strong enough to get through this, too.!" And I thought, "Mom does so well at home; she has lived with Alzheimer's and Vascular Dementia for so long (more than twice as long as expected). If I can get her out of this place and back home, she will live at least several more years."

Then, unfortunately, I switched back to being angry again. This time, I was angry at COVID. I thought, "I wish our wonderful caregivers were here with me to help Mom and me on this lonely and sad night in the ICU." I knew this time they could not come and be with us due to COVID. I thought, "God, please help Mom, and please help me to be stronger." I felt very weak, and Mom was fading, too.

The next morning, day two of living in intensive care, the ICU doctor gave me the results of recent blood tests and a scan. He said things were not looking good. Mom's kidneys were failing. It appears that the c. diff and the sepsis were causing Mom's organs to shut down. Even with her favorite Disney movies playing on the TV, Mom had a very sad and pained face. She continuously had a scary, blank, coma stare, looking out into space. Mom's wonderful personality and smile were nowhere to be seen. I was extraordinarily upset. On my cell phone, I tried again to call the stupid stomach surgeon, the president of the hospital, and hospitalist to help me, somehow, understand how the wrong surgery could have been done to cause all this suffering. Of course, as expected, no one associated with the hospital and this horrible mistake responded.

Every so often I would walk around the hospital, now a Covid ghost town: no guests or family members anywhere. I was feeling sad, too, for the other suffering patients who could not see their families. I tried to recharge myself by praying in the hospital chapel and then walking outside for a little air and sun.

Outside, I felt guilty about walking past angry family members still lined up and trying desperately to see their loved ones inside. I needed to be out of ICU for a few moments to recharge. I asked myself, "Why is this COVID so horrible, and how could COVID have happened to us?"

The cycle of praying, receiving updates from doctors and nurses, holding Mom's hand, and then being mad at myself and the surgeon went on for days. On the morning of the eighth day, one of the ICU doctors told me that Mom looked like she was stabilizing a little. I thought perhaps another miracle was on the way, and I did a little victory dance in my head! In the next breath, this ICU doctor said he wanted to do a tracheotomy on Mom. He said there was a strong risk of a ventilator-induced infection if the ventilator were to stay down Mom's throat too long. He explained that even though a tracheotomy is invasive and leaves a hole in your throat, it would be safer for her.

I thought to myself, "Really? After all Mom's been through, and she is stabilizing, this guy wants to give her a tracheotomy and put a hole in her throat? Now?"

I calmly told the doctor that I wanted to wait on doing a tracheotomy. I reflected on how I jumped too fast doing an invasive feeding tube surgery and wanted to be more conservative this time. I was then shocked because the ICU Doctor, in front of all the nurses in the ICU, started yelling at me! I could not believe it, but he yelled, "Who do you think you are? What kind of son are you? You can't refuse care that your mom needs. You have a lot of nerve!"

I could not believe what I was hearing. Why was I being yelled at? I guess the doctor was one of that special breed of doctors who does not like to being questioned. I could not believe this *stronzo* (a very fitting Italian expletive) young doctor was yelling at me about *my* mother after what she and I had been going through here. Even with no sleep, my anger at the shoemaker surgeon, and my frayed nerves, God and my Italian ancestors protected me (and the doctor) at that moment. I resisted everything I wanted to do and simply ignored this very rude young *stronzo* physician.

On day twelve the assigned ICU physician (not Dr. Stronzo) told me that Mom was continuing to improve. She still needed to stay on the ventilator, but her kidneys were better. The c. dif and sepsis were also a little better, and Mom likely would be ready to go to a rehab facility in a couple of days.

That day I took an hour to look at the two rehab facilities they recommended. I did not like what I saw. With the state of Covid at the time, I knew these places would not let me be with Mom. I knew the reach of my new city council angel friend, Diane Dixon, would not extend to these places. It also looked like there were very few nurses at these places, and I know with COVID my incredible caregivers would not be allowed in to supplement their nursing shortage.

I called the same Director of Home Nursing for the hospital that was so wonderful when Mom needed home nursing a couple months before. I knew care at home would now be even tougher because Mom needed to be on a ventilator and other intensive care equipment. The home nursing director, who before was very optimistic, thought it would be very hard to do this at home. She said she had seen ventilator and ICU-like care at home only once before. My grandmother immediately spoke in my ear from heaven with a gentle but firm voice and said, "If it's been done before, then why can't you do it?"

The Home Nursing Director said she was not able to dispatch home respiratory therapists to manage the ventilator care, but she knew of two places where there were home respiratory therapists who could do this. I made some quick calls and found that you can get a ventilator at home and have respiratory therapists come to the house to manage ventilator care until they could wean Mom off the ventilator. I was beginning to feel good about my plan to get Mom home again. Despite the hospital insisting that bringing Mom home would be unsafe and a bad idea, I knew in my heart that if we could get Mom home stronger and happier, it would be a good thing for her health and wellbeing.

This time, I threw away my decision matrix and instead prayed about this. I was prepared for the extra work and strength I needed to do this. I knew our superstar caregivers would do everything they could to help us at home. I prayed, and I got the answer! I was ready and excited about bringing Mom home. I was just waiting for the hospital to give me the go ahead.

Two days later in the late afternoon, I was sitting holding Mom's hand when out of the blue suddenly Mom started seizing up. Her monitors were beeping and going crazy. The nurses ran in. In the 14 days I had been staying with Mom in the ICU, I had never seen any nurses run. They walked quickly but never ran. I knew something was very wrong. One nurse made a call, and then quickly another group of nurses and a doctor came into Mom's room. Apparently, Mom was having an emergency cardiac problem. I got out of their way, and they worked on Mom. They quickly injected some medicine into her IV and did some electric thing to her heart. After about 20 minutes, Mom's monitors stopped going crazy. The nurses came in to monitor her very frequently for the next few hours. I was so afraid, and I prayed and prayed. I was still hoping Mom could come home soon, but I was worried again. They finally said they suspected some kind of blood clot had triggered this cardiac scare but were not sure. They did some blood work and talked about doing a CT scan later to find out more.

Things were calmer now as night was settling in. The familiar loneliness and night quietness were creeping in. Then, a few hours later, a little after midnight, the buzzers and monitors went crazy again! Again, nurses came running; the cardiac team appeared. Everyone started working on Mom again! I could see this was even worse. This time, they kicked me out of the room altogether. I called Marina and told her things were not good at all, that I thought Mom might be dying and that, COVID rules be damned, she needed to come to the hospital right away!

I waited outside Mom's room in my pale-yellow sanitary COVID gown and mask. I could see a lot of movement through the glass doors into Mom's room. After working frantically behind the glass doors for what seemed like a lifetime, too suddenly and too eerily the frantic movement in the room stopped completely. The doctor then very slowly opened the glass doors and slowly came out of Mom's ICU room. Quiet. Suddenly somber. The doctor slowly took me over to a side area with a small couch and chair. He gestured for me to sit down. Then, he quietly said, "I am very sorry, but your mom did not make it."

I was unpreparedly confused and shocked. My head was spinning. I pulled myself together and said, "I thought Mom was getting better and that we were getting ready to take her home soon." He said sometimes with c. diff and sepsis things can become better and then unexpectedly take a rapid turn for the worse. "How can this be happening?" I asked myself.

The doctor quietly left, and Marina arrived soon after. I told her what the doctor had said, and the two of us just sat on the couch being very sad, quiet, and shocked. We then went back into Mom's room. We stood next to Mom, and we kissed her forehead. I held her hand and cupped her cheek with my other hand. I could feel the warmth of life slowly leave Mom's body. The most vibrant, life-affirming, loving woman on the planet was slowly getting cold and leaving us. Her skin temperature was dropping.

I was at my father's side when he passed more than 30 years before and at my grandmother's side 15 years before. In both cases, I felt the warmth of life leave their bodies, too. You never get used to it. You know when their temperature drops, life as we know it is slowly leaving. With the change of temperature, I could almost feel Mom's spirit and soul lifting as I imagined her watching us hold her hand.

Marina and I just hung out there with Mom, stunned and saddened. In disbelief. We were just about ready to take Mom home. The medical equipment had been reserved, and the skilled nurses were on call. Then this!

Mom passed at about 12:40 am. The most wonderful mom, teacher, and human being on this planet, so full of life and love and passion, was gone soon after Mother's Day in May. Marina and I quietly drove home. We did not know what to say. As those who have experienced this know, seeing your loved one leave you like this is so surreal. I could not believe what had just happened. I cannot describe the emptiness and the big hole in our hearts, especially on this first night when it was so quiet and still at home without Mom. That lonely sad night will stay with me forever.

Chapter Summary

1. C.dif and sepsis are very common killers of the elderly. They are often caused by long-term strong antibiotic therapies. Try not to put your loved one in a position where antibiotics are needed. However, if they need antibiotics try to limit them if possible.

2. With the elderly who have been weakened and have a weak immune system, I learned things can look fine and then apparently take a turn for the worse quickly. Appreciate your loved one when you can. Savor every single moment you have with your loved one now; don't put it off.

3. Suffering and death are never easy. When you feel you are losing strength and hope, pray for strength and pray for your loved one. It will help you, and it will help them.

4. Being your loved one's care leader is so very challenging and also rewarding. It is especially hard in the last phase of their life. That end of the journey is a huge challenge and utterly emotionally draining. At that time, your loved one may not be able to tell you, but they appreciate you very much for taking beautiful care of them. It also doesn't mean the difficult end of life phase grief is not worth the care leader journey. It is an incredible blessing to be a care leader. I know you will do a beautiful job being a care leader, and your loving care will be inspiring.

Loved One Passing:
Grief, Challenges and
New Beginnings

The days after Mom's passing, as some of you have experienced yourselves, were a huge black hole of emptiness. It felt like a new journey was about to begin, but I did not know how or in what direction to even take the first step. The days and weeks immediately after Mom's death felt like a dream state of shock and numbness. I knew I had to focus on being positive and strong to start a new path forward. I tried to think positively and focused on how wonderful Mom was and how she would have wanted me to be happy, even without her. My mind, however, kept drifting back to the hospital horror and Mom's suffering. The hospital stay had been extremely hard, grueling, and terrible for Mom. It was a nightmarishly horrible ending for a mom who deserved a lot more peace and comfort at the end of a remarkable life. Regardless, I had to figure out how to go forward. I felt that I was at the door of something very new and very different. I had no idea what my next chapter would be, but it was coming. Taking care of Mom for so long had been all-consuming, and even though Mom's end was a gut-wrenching nightmare, I had absolutely no regrets about taking this simultaneously wonderfully delightful and challenging (even horrifying at the end) journey through Alzheimer's with Mom.

Counting My Blessings after Mom's Passing

The day after mom passed, Marina and I began the very strange and very difficult baby steps of our new journey. We had to put one foot in front of the other. First, we let our New York family know about Mom's passing. We also informed each of Mom's remarkable caregivers. Finally, we let some of Mom's closest friends know about her passing. Of course, they all wanted to know when the funeral would be. May 2020 was smack in the beginning of the depths of the first wave of Covid. Marina called our church. The woman answering the phone said that due to Covid the priests were not holding any funeral masses. We told the hospital the night mom passed that we wanted Mom buried where my dad and grandmother were buried. The funeral office also said that because of Covid there would be no services until after Covid. After COVID? Would that be a month? Six months? Who knew at the time that COVID would last so long.

Marina, the same thinking-outside-the-box genius who brought you calls to President Trump and the mayor was on another "get an exception to COVID policy" Mission. She called and left a voicemail for our church pastor, Father Steve, asking him to please do a funeral mass for Mom. Father Steve called back later in the day and said he would happily do the funeral mass for Mom as long as our guests were masked, there were not too many people, and we practiced social distancing. Father Steve said that he had not done a funeral mass since Covid started, but he would do it for us. Marina then called the funeral home and told them that if our church pastor was willing to do a full Funeral Mass that it seemed reasonable that the funeral home should be able to do a small, masked and socially distanced service, too. They agreed with that logic. Magic Marina did it again! This was a blessing because Mom went to Catholic School for many years, was deeply dedicated to her faith, and would have wanted that.

Then, we had another blessing. It seems at that time no one wanted to take a COVID risk flying. We totally understood this. Because of this we did not expect any of our New York family would come. Then God blessed us again. Our wonderful cousin, Allison, and her daughter, MacKenzie, took a safer transportation mode (a relatively empty train) from New York to California. The funeral was going to be almost a week away so there was time for them to arrive. We had not seen them for so very long and were very grateful for their love and sacrifice in coming here for Mom and for us.

The funeral service and rosary at the funeral home were beautiful. With a long Alzheimer's journey, most people lose most of their friends. This was especially true for Mom because she also lost her speech very early on, which made staying connected with friends so difficult. Even with Mom' long-term speechless Alzheimer's journey and the depth of COVID, many of Mom's longtime friends came to the funeral. Those who could not come sent dozens of flowers, gifts, cards, and heartfelt condolences. We received many phone calls expressing sorrow and sharing with us lots of amazing long-ago memories of how delightful Mom and their friendship with Mom was. Everyone had so much love and respect for Mom. Of course, each of our five remarkable long-term caregivers came, too.

Everyone close to Mom knew she loved to do adult coloring book drawings during her Alzheimer's journey. As a sign of their love for Mom and to have a loving memento of Mom, I asked each person attending the funeral home service, during the service, to take one of Mom's coloring books and some colored pencils and draw a picture of their choosing in Mom's coloring book. I thought that this was a great way to honor Mom. I also thought Mom would love watching from heaven as each of her guests struggled to draw a picture. Mom was a perfectionist about her drawings, and I'm sure would have improvement suggestions for each of their drawings. I'm also sure Mom, watching from heaven, was very happy that all the people that she loved were coloring in her honor. I, too, enjoyed watching all these people concentrating so hard on their drawings right there in the mortuary chapel. To honor Mom, I insisted they take Mom's coloring book home; they all loved this activity and their wonderful memento of Mom.

Teachers Mom worked with years ago as well as friends from our life long ago in New York and Pomona all reached out for Mom. Even though only a few had had recent contact with Mom, everyone still honored her and loved her. The funeral mass was beautiful. Father Steve did a wonderful job. We are eternally grateful to Father Steve for making an exception for us during Covid to do the funeral mass for us. We were so grateful for everyone who, even in the depths of Covid, came and shared their love, care, and friendship with us. Many of Mom's oldest friends and our wonderful caregivers came to the house after the funeral. All the love and well wishes from so many reminded me and each other how very special Mom was.

Grief: Learning & Healing Actions

Not long after the funeral was over and thank you notes had been sent, an even bigger grief set in for me. I went back to Dr. Lievonen, the therapist I had gone to during Mom's Alzheimer's journey. Dr. Lievonen worked with me on trying to be positive. She wanted me to focus on all the positive memories of Mom. I had no trouble thinking about all about Mom's wonderful qualities. I could also easily think about how well Mom took care of us growing up. I thought of what an amazing teacher she was when I observed her in a classroom with her kindergartners. For holidays, Dr. Lievonen suggested remembering all the wonderful ways Mom would celebrate the holidays. Marina and I frequently went to the cemetery. Going to the cemetery for some reason felt therapeutic. Mom loved birds, and we brought bird houses that Marina hand painted with special notes for Mom written on them and hung them on the tree right next to where Mom and our grandmother were buried together. All these things helped a small amount with our very big grief.

The part of grief that I had the hardest time with, and still have a hard time with occasionally, is reframing the months I lived in the hospital watching Mom suffer so much simply due to that surgeon's horrible medical mistake! This hospital time is the darkest time in my entire life and is still a bit of a block to my fully getting through my grief. The incompetence of the surgeon and my decision to use his services keeps bothering me. I tried to stay grateful that Mom lived longer and happier than anyone expected. I remind myself to be grateful for how happy she was with her five wonderful caregivers and Marina being around her all the time. I reflected on how I was truly grateful for the privilege of being Mom's care leader for so long.

Even with all I had to be grateful for, I was stuck thinking about the surgery mistake and how it led so directly to Mom's death. I thought if I could shift this negative energy to positive action it might help. In my HR role in the corporate world, I taught leaders that positive actions can often transform negative mindsets and their associated behaviors. The idea is that when you act, your mindset and thinking often then align with that action. I decided to take my own advice and channel my negative feelings into positive action.

Turning Grief into Positive Action: Medical Mistakes and the Law

The first big action I took to help with my grief and anger in losing Mom the way I did was to explore a medical negligence lawsuit for Mom's suffering and death. I thought that the doctor doing the exact surgery he said he would not do because it was too dangerous for Mom clearly had to be malpractice.

After some research, I found the four leading medical malpractice law firms in California. I called each of them and shared the story about how the surgeon discovered major stomach scar tissue in a pre-surgery scan, said a stomach G-Tube should not be done due to its danger, and then did the exact G-tube procedure that he said was too dangerous. Then, I told the lawyers how this led to a serious infection, a long surgery to remove the infection, a Grand Canyon surgical wound, months of strong IV antibiotics, leading to c. diff, sepsis, and Mom's death. I told them I had copies of all the records, chart notes, tests, and records they might need.

After I described all this and a little bit about Mom, each of these law firms quickly told me the same thing. They said I had a very strong case for medical malpractice. They said almost certainly that the stomach surgeon would be found medically negligent. Then, in the next breath they all said that even though it is strong case, they would not take it. I asked, "Why won't you take the case if it is so strong?" They said that because Mom was in in her late 80s and had later stage Alzheimer's, the amount of money likely awarded would not be enough to make taking the case worth it for them. I did not understand this if the case was so good.

The attorneys said it was about how damages for medical negligence are calculated. They said damages are based on factors like lost income and pain and suffering. Mom was elderly, not working, and therefore did not have significant lost income. And because of Mom's Alzheimer's and her age, she would have most likely passed in a couple of years, anyway, which limits damages, too. For pain and suffering, they said the defendants would argue that Mom did not suffer all that much incremental pain and suffering because she already was suffering from Alzheimer's. In addition, because California has a cap of $250,000 on medical negligence damages, even if in the unlikely instance that a jury wanted to punish the surgeon and award extra-large punitive damages, the cap was so low there would be little money left over after paying the experts needed to fight the army of people that the doctor, the insurance company, and the hospital would call on to defend the physician.

My head was spinning. As a former HR leader, I knew all about the importance of having incentives and disincentives for work behaviors. I thought what kind of incentive, then, do physicians have to be ultra-careful to protect our elderly if there are no consequences for their medical mistakes? The answer was clear: doctors and hospitals did not have much of an incentive to be ultra-careful with our elderly, especially if they had comorbidities.

I could not believe what I was hearing! I knew that since all these leading law firms were all saying the same thing, elderly patients are in real danger when it comes to medical mistakes. After I realized, I could not realistically sue this shoemaker surgeon, I asked the lawyers about going to the California Medical Board or State Legislature to get this surgeon's license taken away. I could hear laughing in the tone of their voices on the phone. They all told me that trying to get his license taken away would be a huge waste of time. They said the California Medical Board and State Legislature rarely disciplines doctors, and they had never heard of an instance where a doctor had their license taken away. They said, even in the very rare case they discipline a doctor, it takes years to go through the process for this to happen, and all the while the doctor is continuing to practice and very possibly making more grave and tragic medical mistakes. I could not believe what I was hearing. My head started hurting. This was just so wrong on so many levels! How can there not be strong incentives to protect our elderly patients? According to a Johns Hopkins University study, more than 170,000 people die in this country *each year* due directly to medical mistakes. This report noted that 10% of all deaths in this country each year are because of medical error. Another study revealed that nearly half the people in this country have either directly experienced a damaging medical mistake or know someone who did. In California alone, the state board estimates there are five million pharmaceutical mistakes. This is a major crisis; there is a true pandemic of medical errors in this country. Putting strong legal incentives and penalties into place for physicians and hospitals to protect patients would be the required vaccine to stop this pandemic.

Because of this country's tidal wave of medical errors, it is even more important to research the background of your loved one's doctor or surgeon. The first step in looking into the background of your physician is to see what your state medical board or the board of medical examiners has said about this physician. You can find out how long they have been licensed, where they went to medical school, and if the state board has taken any disciplinary action against them. If you are unsure how to locate your state's medical board, you can go to The Federation of State Medical Boards (FSMB), http://www.fsmb.org/. You can also look at local public court records (online) to see if there are malpractice or other kinds of lawsuits against your physician. In addition, if you would like to see other patients' experience with a physician, there are several physician review websites that provide information about years of experience, specialty, hospitals at which they have privileges, and what patients think of the physician. Some of the top physician review sites include Healthgrades, Vitals, RateMDs, and Yelp. In addition to learning to ask great questions of your physician, you should check these websites to dive deeper into the quality of your loved one's physicians. You should also check your loved one's medications. Online websites show photos of what a pill is supposed to look like from each manufacturer. Every pill has etched on it a letter or number. Check the bottle label and the photo of the pill identifier. Nothing is more important than doing your homework on physicians, the hospital, and the medicines to help ensure your loved one does not become another victim of our epidemic of medical errors in this country. It is a little extra work, but it can save your loved one's life.

I mentioned to these malpractice lawyers that I filed a formal complaint with the hospital about what happened. These same lawyers responded to me with a range of interesting reactions like, "don't hold your breath," "good luck with that," and "when hell freezes over." They were right. I never heard back from the hospital, and I know nothing was done because I know this surgeon is still practicing at this hospital. I was profoundly dispirited, but I could not let this go; I still wanted to take positive action in some way.

I called around and networked a little and found the Consumer Watchdog Group in LA that also has a passion for justice and protecting patients. I asked how I could help them with this epidemic of horrible medical mistakes. Consumer Watchdog linked me up with two of their wonderful associates, Michele and Carmen—smart, passionate, experienced women with hearts of gold. They work tirelessly in leading a team of Volunteer Advocates, like me, to fight for Patients' Rights in California. Most of their team of Volunteer Advocates are victims of medical mistakes themselves or have loved ones that were victims of medical mistakes. I joined this powerful little team and have been on many calls with the California Legislature to help fight for patients' rights.

Hearing horrific stories from other victims of medical malpractice was cathartic for me. I learned medical mistakes are unbelievably more common than people know. I learned there is a mountain of money doctors' organizations, hospital organizations, and insurance companies spend every year lobbying State Assemblies and Congress to protect their own rights (as opposed to patients' rights). Because of the amount of money the "medical industrial complex" has to spend, the deck, unfortunately, is stacked against you, me, and our elderly loved ones. Another wonderful trait I learned from both Mom and my grandmother is optimism and belief in people. I may be naïve on this, but I believe we will eventually put the proper incentives and penalties in place to encourage doctors and hospitals to protect patients much better than they do today. It will take more time, more money, and most important, more courageous and inspirational leaders in our state and federal legislatures and in our medical corporations—and more media exposure. I am optimistic because I know people like Michele and Carmen from Consumer Watchdog who, like me and my fellow volunteer advocates, will not give up on this literally life and death issue.

Turning Grief into Action: UCI MIND

I was talking to Linda, the wonderful Director of Development at UCI MIND at UC Irvine, shortly after Mom passed. I was talking to her about some of the things I did to take care of Mom at home. She told me what I did taking care of her at home with Alzheimer's was terrific and that I had really learned a lot. She said that UCI MIND was doing a podcast series on dementia caregiving called *Spotlight on Care*, and asked if I might be interested in doing some podcasts about home care in this series? I thought this was another great way to take action to soothe my grief and at the same time, help others learn from my experience. Linda linked me up with an empathetic woman named Virginia, who was co-hosting with Steve a UCI MIND podcast series on dementia caregiving. I did a couple podcasts and really enjoyed doing them. Because Mom went to the UCI MIND Alzheimer's Center for her diagnosis and ongoing care with one of her terrific neurologists, I feel a real affinity to work with UCI MIND as much as I can. Everyone associated with UCI MIND is exceptionally passionate, talented, and diligent in helping dementia patients and their families.

Encouragement from Virginia, Steve, and people who listened to my podcasts gave me the confidence to consider writing a book about what I had learned as a care leader. Also, after listening to my podcasts, Linda, the director, saw my passion for helping others with Alzheimer's care and asked me to join UCI MIND's Advisory Board. It has been a distinct honor to work for such an important cause with so many incredible people. Virginia, Linda, Steve, and others on the UCI MIND team have been a real blessing to me as friends and partners and have helped me take positive action that is helping with my ongoing grief. I am deeply grateful for UCI MIND.

More Wonderful Blessings

Another blessing that came from Mom and our Alzheimer's journey is a continuing friendship with all five of Mom's superpowered caregivers. We share birthdays and special events. They all still are part of our family—each of them, who in their unique and special way, took loving care of Mom, displaying compassion, creativity, and a range of talents Their care was much better than I could ever have imagined or hoped for. They were also there for us, whether it was at home or staying with Mom in those dark days in the hospital. Their love, skills, and commitment were an inspiration and a blessing to us then and now.

I am also unbelievably grateful for my sister Marina! Marina's ability to think outside the box enabled me to be in the hospital through the depths of Mom's dark suffering during Covid when no guests were allowed. Marina was my MVP 6th man (woman) of the year, assistant manager, facilities manager, energizer, and glue on Championship Team Mom. More than that, we would not be able to get through our grief without leaning on each other.

After experiencing Mom's horrific suffering in the hospital, I don't like the idea of going to a hospital myself. Fear of going to a hospital filled with Covid patients during the pandemic made us extra careful. Marina and I essentially quarantined ourselves for the entire Covid stretch. Friends of ours who know that Marina and I differ in many ways wondered how we would survive being quarantined together during Covid for so long. The explanation? Marina and I share core values, inculcated by Mom, like the importance of family, faith, empathy, and passion for what is right and just. Both our differences and our similarities helped make us good co-leaders of Mom's care. Great sports or business leaders know that just enough similarities and just enough differences are the ingredients of a championship team. Our similarities bonded us, and our differences made our care for Mom better. Marina and I grow even closer as we continue to support each other through our grief and into our new life journey.

You may have trouble getting along with a sibling or other family members. If you focus on your similar values and the grace God has given you, you will be able to put your ego and pride aside long enough to get along better in order to help your loved one. Family is a great gift from God. Whether coping with something as devastating as Alzheimer's or just working together for a family member needing help, family bonds invoke power. Involving family in the holy moments of beautifully taking care of your loved one with dementia can help your family rise above past grievances. With family help, you can better take care of your loved one with Alzheimer's or any other medical or other problem your family encounters. You can reap the benefits of relationships with family during your loved one's dementia journey and potentially long after. Whether your loved one with dementia is still with you or not, they would want you to be close to and love your whole family always.

Forever Grateful for Mom

Finally, I cannot express enough gratitude for my special mother. The list of gifts Mom gave me is unending. These Mom gifts include strong values, my faith, love, a good education, skills, courage, determination, great life experiences, positivity, confidence, and more. If it were not for these gifts, I could never have been the successful care leader I tried to be. Nor would I be the person I strive to be today. I was so blessed and privileged to be able to spend many magnificent years with Mom before and during her Alzheimer's journey. Said simply, I owe everything I am, everything I have, and everything I will be to Mom. I could not in a million years express all the gratitude I have for my mother.

Chapter Summary

1. Medical mistakes occur much more commonly than people realize. Be hyper alert to this. Watch your loved one's medical team like a hawk, especially if there is surgery involved. Check out the surgeon and hospital carefully. The resources section

of this book contains suggestions on how to check out your medical team.

2. Losing your loved one after a long, grueling emotional, dementia journey is very, very hard. The grief can be overwhelming. Going to an individual therapist or grief group can be immensely valuable. There is nothing weak about getting help with your grief. Some sources for help can be found in the resource section.

3. If you do not work through it, your grief can easily stay with you, leading to physical or psychological problems. People who don't work through their grief can experience dizziness, panic, and other physical and emotional ailments.

4. Try also taking positive actions to help you with grief. Consider aligning some of these positive actions with a way to honor your deceased loved one. This could include mending relationships with family members, volunteering with dementia organizations, or helping causes your loved one had passion for.

Conclusion

Leading your loved one's care is very challenging; it can be physically and emotionally exhausting. Yet, it is also a wonderful blessing and a gift. Your loved one can thrive with your loving care leadership. You will see all your love, your capabilities, and the energy that make up you come together to make a huge difference for your loved one in the time in their life where they need you the very most. Alzheimer's or any dementia must be unbelievably scary for a loved one. They need you now more than ever! You can be their superhero and be there for them in their darkest hour.

As you reflect on all my dementia care leadership learning and this Alzheimer's love story, I know you will have a lot to think about. Breakthrough care categories of actions, leadership tools, mindset changes, barriers to overcome, and lots of resources and aids are provided here to help you. If you feel a little overwhelmed by these things or caring for your loved one overall, remember: if you peel it all back, at the very core of care is simply love. Your love will pour over you, empowering and compelling you to make things as good for your loved one as you can possibly imagine them to be. All these breakthrough care pillars and their leadership derive their energy and power from your love. Your creatively compassionate core and the extended care team you will lead all derive their superpowers from your best superpower, your love, and its associated willingness to sacrifice for your loved one. It is less about starting out with superhuman care leader skills as it is about having a superhuman heart. Your interest in reading this book and considering taking these actions to extend the life, health, and happiness of your loved one tells me you have a superhuman heart.

Turning your empowering love into positive actions so your loved one lives longer and happier is the noblest mission there is. There is nothing more noble and rewarding than this. As you create your own Alzheimer's or dementia love story, here are a few questions designed to help turn your desire into positive actions.

I am a care leader who ___________________________________

I want to be a care leader who___________________________________

Internal conflicts that are in my way include___________________________________

Actions I need to take to overcome conflicts and be the care leader I want to be include ___________________________________

Attitudes I will need to have are___________________________________

Remind yourself of all you have done in your life and all you are capable of. This will bolster your self-esteem and empower you to follow your dreams.

If you activate this Breakthrough Care System, know that it will help your loved one so much! I tried to bring the best care leadership I could to every encounter and touchpoint that my mom had. I had to learn everything on the job, but that did not discourage me. I felt compelled to help Mom in the way I did simply because I loved her.

What I did helped Mom live healthier, longer and happier, but I am sure it could have been done even better. Improving on these care actions or coming up with your own even more powerfully creative breakthrough care actions would be so great! To get even bolder and bigger results for your loved one, you are only limited by: 1) the depth of your love and super-powered passion to help your loved one live longer, healthier, and happier; 2) your drive to find, lead, motivate, and retain the finest creatively compassionate care team ever; and 3) you and your care team's willingness to learn and try taking even more innovative creatively compassionate care actions.

As you saw from the chapters about my mom in the hospital, I made mistakes. You might even make a mistake or two in your care leadership. Humans, and physicians too, make mistakes. Doing the very best you can to help your loved one is what is important. Your loved one will know and appreciate you for the loving and empowered care you provide. Anxiety and dementia may prevent them from showing you their gratitude. However, know they love you and appreciate you. Be peacefully confident that what you are doing for your loved one is noble even if you don't hear their gratitude. This long dementia journey with your loved one is your and their ultimate love story. In fact, the deep commitment and sacrifice that is care leadership is the definition of love. There is no greater love than the sacrifice this takes. When love is easy, it can still be love, but this kind of love is hard and takes digging deep inside yourself to bring out the best there is in you. The marathon of dementia care is a huge act of love.

I was certainly blessed to experience many holy moments in Mom's long Alzheimer's journey. Sure, it was the most intellectually, emotionally, and physically challenging thing I have ever done. At the same time, it is the most important, rewarding, and inspiring thing I have ever done, too. My hope is that you will receive the same remarkable gift and the same rewarding experience I had. I know you will help your loved one live longer, healthier and happier. Remember the wise words of my incredible Sicilian grandmother who is speaking with you right now from heaven: "If my grandson can do this, you can, too (and possibly even better)!" If we find a cure for Alzheimer's and dementia, that would be awesome; but our loved ones can't wait. We must act powerfully and boldly immediately on the many small things within our control that collectively can be done to make a big difference for them. We must be empowered care leaders for our loved ones right now!

Resources for Empowered Care Leaders

Achieving Breakthroughs

Clear, J. (2018). Atomic habits: Tiny changes, remarkable results. Avery.

Dweck, C. S. (2016). Mindset: The new psychology of success. Ballantine Books.

O'Keeffe, J. (1998). Business beyond the box: Applying your mind for breakthrough results. Nicholas Brealey Publishing.

Understanding the Brain & Dementia

Attia, P. (2023). *Outlive: The science and art of longevity.* Harmony Books.

Bredesen, D. E. (2020). *The end of Alzheimer's: The first program to prevent and reverse cognitive decline.* Avery.

Gupta, S. (2021). *Keep sharp: Build a better brain at any age.* Simon & Schuster.

Recharging Passion and Purpose

Kelly, M. (2022). *Holy moments.* Blue Sparrow.

Robinson, K. (2013). *Finding your element: How to discover your talents & passions and transform your life.* Penguin Books.

Alzheimer's and Dementia Care General Know How Building

Alzheimer's Association. (n.d.). *Educational classes.* https://www.alz.org

Attia, P. (2023). *Outlive: The science and art of longevity.* Harmony Books.

Basting, A. (2021). *Creative care: A revolutionary approach to dementia and elder care.* HarperOne.

Bredesen, D. E. (2020). *The end of Alzheimer's: The first program to prevent and reverse cognitive decline.* Avery.

Forester, B., & Harrison, T. (2022). *The complete family guide to dementia: Everything you need to help your parent and yourself.* The Guilford Press.

Graff-Radford, J., & Lund, A. (2020). *Mayo Clinic on Alzheimer's disease & other dementias.* Mayo Clinic Press.

Gupta, S. (2021). *Keep sharp: Build a better brain at any age.* Simon & Schuster.

Knowles, M. S. (1975). *Self-directed learning: A guide for learners and teachers.* Association Press.

Mace, N. L., & Rabins, P. V. (2021). *The 36-hour day: A family guide to caring for people who have Alzheimer disease and other dementias.* Johns Hopkins University Press.

Weatherill, G. (2020). *The caregiver's guide to dementia: Practical advice for caring for yourself and your loved one.* Rockridge Press.

Wisniewski, M. (2019). *Caregiving both ways: A guide for caring for a loved one with dementia (and yourself!).* Mango Media.

Leading Yourself and Leading a Care Team

Hill, A., & Wooden, J. (2001). *Be quick—but don't hurry: Finding success in the teachings of a lifetime.* Simon & Schuster.

Novak, D. (2012). *Taking people with you: The only way to make things happen*. Penguin Group.

Ratliff, J. (2020). *Leadership through trust & collaboration*. Morgan James Publishing.

Zenger, J., & Folkman, J. (2002). *The extraordinary leader: Turning good managers into great leaders*. McGraw-Hill.

Overcoming the Financial Barrier

The National Consumer Voice for Quality Long Term Care
https://theconsumervoice .org/uploads

Olson. S. (2018). *Simple LTC Solution*. Independently Published.

Overcoming Resentment and the Psychological Barrier

Davis, P. (2021). *Floating in the deep end: How caregivers can see beyond Alzheimer's*. Liveright Publishing.

Westfall, J. (2012). *Getting past what you'll never get over: Help for dealing with life's hurts*. Revell Publishing.

Overcoming the Time Barrier

Lakein, A. (1989). *How to get control of your time and your life*. Signet.

Tracy, B. (2017). *Eat that frog: 21 great ways to stop procrastinating and get more done in less time*. Berrett-Koehler.

Overcoming the Self-confidence Barrier

Bonham-Carter, D. (2016). *Building self-esteem: A five-point plan for valuing yourself more*. Icon Books.

Jeffers, S. (1987). *Feel the fear and do it anyway*. Fawcett Columbine.

Loehr, J. E. (1994). *Toughness training for life*. Plume Publishing.

Renewing and Reenergizing Yourself

Abbitt, L. (2017). *The conscious caregiver: A mindful approach to caring for your loved one without losing yourself.* Adams Media.

Colman Mitchell, D. (2020). *Four-quadrant living: A guide to nourishing your mind, body, relationships, and environment.* Four Quadrant Media.

Samples, P., Larsen, D., & Larsen, M. (2000). *Self-care for caregivers: A twelve-step approach.* Hazelden Publishing.

Senn, L. (2017). *The mood elevator: Take charge of your feelings & become a better you.* Berrett-Koehler Publishers.

Getting Help and Support

Alzheimer's Association. (n.d.). Educational classes; support groups; 24x7 hour help line; adult day care centers. https://www.alz.org

Ostrowski, P. (2020). It's not that simple: Helping families navigate the Alzheimer's journey. Self-published.

Psychology Today. (n.d.). Find a therapist. https://www.psychologytoday.com

Ensuring a Safe Environment

Alzheimer's Association. (n.d.). *Home safety checklist.*
https://www.alz.org/media/Documents/
alzheimers-dementia-safety-checklist-ts.pdf

Huff, J. (2023). *Secure spaces: A caregiver's journal and guide to dementia safety at home.* Independently Published.

Town, L., & Kassel, K. (2019). *Home safety checklist and guide for medication safety, driving, and wandering.* Independent Publishing.

Selecting Great People

Kador, J. (1997). *The manager's book of questions: Great interview questions for hiring the best person.* McGraw-Hill.

Coaching, Motivating, and Retaining Remarkable People

Hargrove, R. (1995). *Masterful coaching: Extraordinary results by impacting people and the way they think and work together.* Jossey-Bass.

Kouzes, J. M., & Posner, B. Z. (2003). *Encouraging the heart: A leader's guide to rewarding and recognizing others.* Jossey-Bass.

Mager, R. F., & Pipe, P. (1997). *Analyzing performance problems.* Pitman Learning.

Creating Fun, Stimulating, and Comforting Dementia Experiences (Environment & People)

Brenner, T., & Brenner, K. (2019). *The Montessori method for connecting to people with dementia.* Jessica Kingsley Publishers.

Huebner, B., & Lange, D. (2011). *I remember better when I paint; art & Alzheimer's: Opening doors, making connections.* Bethesda Communications.

Photozig, Inc. (n.d.-a). *Caring response for caregivers* [Mobile app]. Google Play Store. https://play.google.com/store/apps/details?id=com.photozig.caringresponse

Photozig, Inc. (n.d.-b). *Dementia caring response* [Mobile app]. Apple App Store. https://apps.apple.com/us/app/dementia-caring-response/id1314737683

Shouse, D. (2016). *Connecting in the land of dementia: Creative ideas to explore together.* Central Recovery Press.

Wayman, L. (2011). *A loving approach to dementia care: Making meaningful connections with the person who has Alzheimer's disease or other dementia or memory loss.* Johns Hopkins University Press.

Building Medical Knowledge

Reputable Medical Sites: pubmed.ncbi;mayoclinic.org; myclevelandclinic.org; webmd.com

Finding Physician Gurus: Medical School Specialty Departments at Major Universities.

Working Effectively with Your Loved One's Doctor

Berger, Z. D. (2013). *Talking to your doctor: A patient's guide to communicating in the exam room and beyond.* Rowman & Littlefield.

Groopman, J. (2007). *How doctors think.* Houghton Mifflin Company.

Brain and Body Healthy Nutrition

Andrews, J. (2020). *The brain healthy cookbook: MIND diet recipes to prevent disease and enhance cognitive power.* Rockridge Press.

Balch, P. A. (2004). *Prescription for nutritional healing: A-to-Z guide to supplements.* Avery.

Weil, A. (2005). *Healthy aging: A lifelong guide to your physical and spiritual well-being.* Knopf.

Research nutrition, supplements, medicines: *pubmed.ncbi;mayoclinic.org; myclevelandclinic.org; webmd.com*

Avoiding Medical Mistakes

Federation of State Medical Boards. (n.d.). *FSMB: State medical boards.* http://www.fsmb.org/

Healthgrades. (n.d.). *Physician reviews.* https://www.healthgrades.com/

Local court records. (n.d.). *Public access to malpractice and other lawsuits.* [State or county-specific websites vary].

RateMDs. (n.d.). *Physician reviews.* https://www.ratemds.com/

Vitals. (n.d.). *Physician reviews.* https://www.vitals.com/

Yelp. (n.d.). *Physician reviews.* https://www.yelp.com/

Making Good Decisions & Avoiding Care Decision Errors

Russo, J. E., & Schoemaker, P. J. H. (2002). *Winning decisions: Getting it right the first time.* Doubleday.

Working through Grief for Your Loved One

Devine, M. (2017). *It's ok that you're not ok: Meeting grief and loss in a culture that doesn't understand.* Sounds True.

Kessler, D. (2020). *Finding meaning: The sixth stage of grief.* Scribner.

Reference List

Americans' experiences with medical errors and patient safety. (2017). NORC at the University of Chicago and IHI/NPSF Lucian Leape Institute.

Carbone, L. (2004). *Clued in: How to keep customers coming back again and again*. FT Press.

Clear, J. (2018). *Atomic habits: Tiny changes, remarkable results*. Avery.

Davis, P. (2021). *Floating in the deep end: How caregivers can see beyond Alzheimer's*. Liveright Publishing.

Granneman, J., & Solo, A. (2024). *Sensitive: The hidden power of the highly sensitive person*. Harmony Press.

Gupta, S. (2021). *Keeping sharp: Build a better brain at any age*. Simon & Schuster.

Jeffers, S. (1987). *Feel the fear and do it anyway*. Fawcett Columbine.

Kelly, M. (2022). *Holy moments*. Blue Sparrow.

Lives lost: An updated comparative analysis of avoidable deaths in hospitals each year. (2019). Johns Hopkins School of Medicine.

National Institutes of Health. (2011, September). *Sedative load of medications prescribed for older people with dementia in care homes*. PubMed.

O'Keeffe, J. (1998). *Business beyond the box: Applying your mind for breakthrough results*. Nicholas Brealey Publishing.

Oxford University Press. (n.d.). Going gets tough, the tough get going, when the. In *The Oxford Dictionary of Phrase and Fable. Retrieved August 25, 2025, from Oxford Reference.*

Senn, L. (2017). *The mood elevator: Take charge of your feelings and become a better you.* Berrett-Koehler Publishers.

About the Author

Mark Wilson had a long career as a human resources leader for Fortune 500 Companies, including more than 20 years leading Leadership and Organization Effectiveness for Taco Bell, a PepsiCo then YUM! Brands company.

Mark decided to leave his leadership development and human resources career to stay home to take care of his mother who developed Alzheimer's. This is their journey of how he applied many of the leadership practices he learned in his career to leading his mom's care. Mark shows how these leadership practices helped him lead his mother's care in a way that led to her living longer and happier than anyone expected. His dedication to help his mom led to discovering this breakthrough care system. These breakthrough care pillars are powerful and are dependent on empowered care leadership to activate them in a way that leads to breakthrough results in longevity and happiness.

Mark has done podcasts for the UCI MIND Alzheimer's Center and other leading organizations. He is on the Advisory Board for the UCI MIND Center and serves as a Volunteer Advocate for the Consumer Watchdog Group working to reduce medical errors and champion patients' rights in California. Mark also leads several Alzheimer's Family Support Groups for the Alzheimer's Association and is on the Alzheimer's Legislative Advocacy Team for the Alzheimer's Association.